EMPOWERED CHOICES

A Guide to Healing Head & Neck Pain

DANIELLE MALLETT

Copyright © 2023 by Danielle Mallett

All rights reserved. No part of this publication may be reproduced, distributed, or transmitted in any form or by any means, including photocopying, recording, or other electronic or mechanical methods, without the prior written permission of the publisher, except in the case of brief quotations embodied in critical reviews and certain other noncommercial uses permitted by copyright law.

Printed in the United States of America- First Edition

ISBN: 9780999191736

Edited by Louise Place
Illustrated by Ian Walker

Visit us online @:
getwellwithdanielle.com

Credit to the Monterey Peninsula Writers Group. I couldn't have finished this book without all of your help!

*This book is dedicated to dreamers, creatives,
disembodied souls interested in befriending their body,
all the loved ones lost to suicide, my fiance, my children,
my siblings, my family and friends who raised me, and to
8-year-old me who never gave up on her dream to be a writer.*

OTHER BOOKS BY DANIELLE MALLETT

Fiction
Take Me Away with You

Poetry
Sunshine by Design

TABLE OF CONTENTS

HEAD AND NECK INJURIES

Introduction ix

Chapter 1 Concussion 1

Chapter 2 Whiplash 19

Chapter 3 Depression 29

STEPS TO HEAL HEAD AND NECK PAIN

Chapter 4 Steps to Heal Head and Neck Pain 39

Chapter 5 Feel-Good Relief Tips 53

Chapter 6 Identify Good vs. Bad Pain 61

Chapter 7 Exercises for Head and Neck Health 67

Chapter 8 Find a Healing Professional 119

RESOURCES AND REMINDERS

Chapter 9 Empowered Choices for Specific Neck Pain 131

Chapter 10 Before You Go 141

Chapter 11 Massage Resources 145

Chapter 12 Movement Resources 155

Bibliography 161

INTRODUCTION

It happened in a busy Trader Joe's parking lot. I fainted from dehydration and menstrual cramps. My head hit the gravel the way a bowling ball drops onto a lane. I was knocked unconscious, went into a seizure, and was rushed to the hospital where they treated me for internal bleeding.

This head injury back in 2004 was the catalyst that got me interested in learning how to heal my head and neck pain, so I could help others heal too. I had accumulated many injuries in my youth—a cracked collarbone, whiplash, concussions, and a shoulder misalignment—but this traumatic brain injury made the head and neck pain I was living with unbearable.

Looking back, I wish I had a resource to help me navigate what was working and what wasn't. There was a lot of trial and error, which was to be expected, but with some guidance, I'm confident I could have healed sooner. That's why I became a Functional Movement Coach; Personal Trainer, Massage, and CranioSacral Therapist—and why I wrote this book. Drawing from my own personal battles and struggles, *Empowered Choices: A Guide to Healing Head & Neck Pain* is full of useful information on how to better cope, remedy, and heal from head and neck pain. I wrote it to empower you to become your own healer. Chances are you have endured pain for a long time. I believe the only way to truly heal is to become an active participant in the process of healing.

After earning my bachelor's degree from Naropa University, I worked to become a certified yoga teacher with a focus in yoga therapy, a California certified massage and CranioSacral therapist, a certified National Academy of Sports Medicine personal trainer, and most recently a certified Foundation Training instructor. For eight years, I have coached clients to gain stability, mobility, and strength with my business—*Get Well with Danielle*.

It took years of learning about the body through yoga, massage, and CranioSacral Therapy before I found Foundation Training, the final puzzle piece to healing my head and neck pain. Ultimately, it was a combination of these modalities that got my body to a place of peace. Though the puzzle pieces to your healing may be different, this book will help you find what you need faster.

Have you suffered a concussion or whiplash? Is your neck weak or stiff? Do you lack mobility or feel pain after using technology too much? Are you a new mom with neck pain from staring down at your adorable baby? Have you tried to improve your situation by going to doctors, chiropractors, yoga classes, massage therapists, or personal trainers—only to still be in pain and feel dejected? If yes, I understand. Rest assured: I have been where you are and come out the other side. This book, full of new options, is for you.

Do you feel stuck because you're not sure where to start? Or did you try one thing only to find it didn't work and then lose momentum or hope? This book will give you practical tools to help you move out of pain. Do you struggle with the motivation to exercise because some days even simple movements, such as getting into the car and looking over your shoulder, are difficult? I made this book for you.

INTRODUCTION

Section 1: Head and Neck Injuries covers a range of upper body injuries. Chapter 1 and 2 address two common head and neck injuries: concussions and whiplash. I share what happened when I experienced these injuries and explain basic anatomy of the head, neck, and shoulders to offer an understanding of what can go wrong with these injuries. The more you understand, the easier it will be for you to decide which modality will help most. Chapter 3 talks about depression, a common and often unknown side effect of a traumatic brain injury. Each chapter ends with one or two healing puzzle pieces that helped me and can help you too.

Section 2: The Four Steps to Heal Head and Neck Pain offers a practical breakdown with manageable steps. You'll learn ways to relieve your pain, identify good vs. bad pain, and exercises to practice. I'll also show you how to find a healing professional, how to decide who to work with, and which questions to ask once you're working with the chosen practitioner.

Section 3: Resources and Reminders guides you toward making empowered choices for your specific neck pain. I cover various types of head and neck pain that come from previous injuries, too much technology, being a new mom, and more. We revisit all of the steps you can take to heal. Finally, chapters 11 and 12 break down the types of massage & movement resources available to you.

Simple, straightforward, and safe, the exercises in this book will increase stability, mobility, and strength in your neck, and, as a result, your head and neck pain will diminish. You'll learn about the movements that hurt your head and neck, and the ones that make it stronger.

Use this book in the way that works best for you. Think of it as a Choose Your Own Adventure. It doesn't have to be read from beginning to end. If my personal stories are helpful and interesting, then by all means read them, but know that all the resources are here for you to find them as quickly as possible. You can flip through to use it as a reference guide and review the healing puzzle pieces at the end of each chapter. Then when you find a healing puzzle piece that sounds helpful, such as CranioSacral Therapy, skip ahead to the suggested chapter to find more information.

However you approach this book, my hope is that you use it to feel informed and empowered with the choices you're making to heal your head and neck pain.

MY HEAD AND NECK PAIN

In 2003, I went to college in Boulder, Colorado and realized three things:

1. **I couldn't do a sit-up.**
   I remember lying on the grass with a group of friends, and when it was time to get up, I had to roll over on my side to push up to a seated position. At the time, I had severe neck pain from previous concussions, whiplash, and overall physical weakness.

2. **I struggled with yoga.**
   I spent most yoga classes mentally comparing myself to the able-bodied people in the room. I hated my body, especially my neck, wrists, and lower back, because of my reoccurring pain. I was convinced that plank, downward dog, and many of the standing postures in yoga were created to torture people. It took years to develop a practice that felt good.

3. **I had limited body awareness.**
   When faced with mindfulness and wisdom of the body classes, I felt awkward, out of touch, and not equipped to

INTRODUCTION

handle the inner feelings that arose. I resisted befriending a body I'd spent years disliking. The only time I was aware of my body was when it was in excruciating pain. I learned to live with chronic neck pain. The only relief I got was from chiropractic neck adjustments and massages, but the pain always returned after a few weeks. It was infuriating. I was too young to feel that out of shape.

I became determined to answer two questions: Where was the pain coming from, and how could I get rid of it—permanently?

CHAPTER 1

CONCUSSION

A concussion is also called a minor traumatic brain injury. A minor traumatic brain injury! Why isn't that talked about more? An injury to the brain is a big deal, even if it's minor. Concussions happen all the time in sports, car accidents, and everyday incidents. The thing about concussions is that the pain isn't always felt right away. Plus, symptoms not only vary, but also may take a few days, or even weeks, to recognize.

Anyone who has had a concussion knows how disorienting it can be. It's common to experience fatigue. It is difficult to know if the exhaustion is coming from the concussion or from everyday strain, especially if you experienced a concussion early in life. When I had a concussion as a child, I remember feeling tired and confused. I remember struggling with mood changes. I thought that was part of growing up. What I didn't realize was that the damage caused to the brain from multiple concussions is invisible from the outside. A concussion can damage blood vessels, injure nerves, and cause depression. Symptoms to look out for: headaches, nausea, fatigue, confusion, memory problems, sleep disturbances, and/or mood changes.

After a concussion, it's important to take it easy. Limit any activity that adds to your symptoms. Maybe it's too much computer or television--screen time can aggravate symptoms. Maybe it's talking on the phone or being under bright lights. Pay attention to what you're feeling, and give your brain time to heal by doing less. All brain injuries, even minor concussions, will slow you down, and it's important to not rush the healing process. Just because you don't have internal bleeding or a broken bone doesn't mean you aren't experiencing a wide range of symptoms. Be gentle with your body as your brain heals.

If you experience a concussion while playing sports, it's important to get cleared before you return to them, so you don't risk a second concussion, which is more likely if you're still having headaches, or feeling dizzy, disoriented, or confused.

In the stories below, you'll learn about the luckless ways I experienced concussions and discover the puzzle pieces I found to heal.

TRAUMATIC BRAIN INJURY

In my early twenties, after a day of running into gas station bathrooms with wedding cake diarrhea, horrible menstrual cramps, and nausea, I dragged myself to the passenger side of my friend's car in a Trader Joe's parking lot. The car door was locked. Everything around me started to spin. My cramps intensified. Before I could kneel down, everything went black.

The next moment, bells jingled, and I saw myself wrapped in angel wings. My eyes shot open, ready to see the after-life. At first there were white lights, but they weren't heavenly, as I'd imagined they would be.

CHAPTER 1: CONCUSSION

Instead, they were fluorescent shining on my friend who was standing beside my hospital bed with a flip phone. Her hands were shaking as she asked, "Danielle, what's your dad's number?" The white walls of the Intensive Care Unit matched her pale face.

Someone tugged at my hair. "We're going to have to shave it."

Crap, if I live through this, will I be bald? Is that really my first thought upon waking up? How vain am I? What if I don't live? What if this is it? I focused on my friend's brown eyes and avoided her shaking hands. *How serious is this?*

I wanted to close my eyes and disappear, but I kept them open and recited my dad's number,, "7-0-2 … I have to pee," I whispered. Almost immediately, a catheter was inserted, causing a sharp pain between my legs. My body jolted from the abrupt placement, and then I went unconscious again for what felt like seconds, but in actuality was over an hour.

I was transferred to an ambulance to take me to a hospital for patients with severe head trauma. I had internal bleeding, and the second hospital was better equipped to determine where the bleeding was coming from. The paramedics eased my gurney out of the ambulance and let it drop several inches to the pavement. The jolt and bright outdoor light forced my eyes open. A paramedic put their hand on my arm and said, "They're more aggressive at this hospital. Be prepared." They seemed to float above me like an angel. I was still convinced this was the end of my life, and I was on my way to heaven. That was before I found out what the angel meant by "more aggressive."

Inside, the nurses slid a stiff board under my body and transported me from the patient room to CAT scans to monitor the subdural hematoma (a fancy way of saying there was internal bleeding in my head). Then I fell into a coma, which is common for this condition. They monitored me closely to make sure I wasn't getting worse and that they didn't need to do surgery. This lasted a few days, and all I remember is being transferred like a limp doll from room to room. Then the internal bleeding stopped.

A couple of days later, I woke up alone, in a dark room, with a needle in one arm and my blood-crusted scalp scratching against a pillow. It felt as if tiny bugs were crawling under my skin from the morphine drip. I wanted to scream for someone to take it out, but the drugs were tranquilizing. I could see the world around me, but I couldn't participate in it. I'm not sure how many days I spent in the hospital, but in order to leave I knew I had to prove I could walk. I was led to a set of stairs and told to walk up them. This was the first time I used my recently acquired meditative practices I was learning in college at Naropa University. It took all of my concentration to see beyond the blurry staircase.

To this day, I remember looking down at my feet and at the bottom step, and saying to myself, "One step at a time, that's all I have to do." The next thing I knew, I had made it up the staircase and back down. That is all any of us can do: take one step at a time. Why is it so easy to forget this?

NEW BODY

In the coming days, I had trouble remembering what I said. I slurred my words, spoke slowly, and repeated myself. I had dizzy spells and no energy. I had to be driven around, and all I wanted to do was sleep. My brain was swollen, and I felt far from healthy.

The short-term internal bleeding, coma, and recovery was a wake-up call. I realized I knew nothing about my anatomy: how

CHAPTER 1: CONCUSSION

it worked, why it was hurting, how to help myself. My hips felt like foreign objects attached to my body, but very far from my brain. My arms and legs felt like they weren't connected to my torso. On the outside, I had a fully functioning body. It didn't look like anything was wrong, besides my delayed speech, which could be chalked up to the drugs and brain swelling. But on the inside, I felt stuck with a broken body at age 21.

After my accident, I was eager to return to my fall semester at Naropa University and get back into the strong home yoga practice I'd developed in Boulder. The doctors said I couldn't fly in a plane for a few weeks because the airplane pressure could damage areas of the brain that were healing, so my dad and aunt drove us past cornfields and over state lines, stopping only for food and sleep. I was on Lortabs for the pain.

When I arrived home, I rolled out my yoga mat to practice, but nothing in my body or mind was the same. My body was weak and in pain. My brain was slow, depressed, and foggy. The yoga practice I'd built up to was gone and replaced with a lot of lying on my back. I rested in gentle twists and felt overcome with nausea, a common side effect of brain trauma. I couldn't move quickly from side to side because the fluids in my brain shifted, making me dizzy and nauseous. I stayed in the twists for long periods and gave my body time to relax. I waited for the spinning in my head to settle and witnessed the nauseous sensations lessening.

At the time, my head hurt so bad that I didn't even notice the left side of my body felt numb. The dizziness and pain in my head held all of my attention. By the time I worked my way back to holding tougher positions, such as downward-facing dog, lunges, and warrior poses, I was in pain everywhere. I didn't know why or where any of the pain was coming from. All I knew was that it didn't take much movement to exhaust me. I was chronically tired.

Nothing felt the same. It took years before the left side of my body started to function properly without pain. In minor ways, it's still delayed, but I no longer expect perfection. I am grateful to live most days without head and neck pain. I have learned to accept this new body and acknowledge that all of the tools in this book are available to you because of the healing that came after this injury.

I hope that the physical pain and limitations you're experiencing lessen over time and that you keep an open mind as you discover what works best for your healing. Remember: it takes time and patience to retrain your new body. Approach it with curiosity, and healing will follow. Here's a quick exercise to remind you that every body has limitations and separating your old body from your new body can help give your power back.

HEALING PUZZLE PIECE
#1 - Wisdom of the Body

With each step on the healing journey, I have learned to listen to the wisdom of my body. At first, this concept was foreign to me. I grew up with my body, but it was something I only paid attention to when it was sick or in pain. It had never occurred to me to listen to my body for any other reason.

The first time I was confronted with this concept was during my first yoga class back in 2001 before yoga was the craze it is today. I was a senior in high school, and I remember having to fight the judgmental voice in my head that believed, "Yoga was boring, and yoga people were weird!" I placed my used exercise mat between two people and watched as more and more students flooded in. People were lined mat to mat; some even set up yoga mats on the deck outside of the studio. This female instructor was popular. It was a huge production. I would

CHAPTER 1: CONCUSSION

have chickened out and left, but that meant wading through at least 50 people. My introvert wasn't having it. The only way out was to brave the class. I was trapped, so I went with it.

Ten minutes into class, I was dripping sweat and worried I might faint. Sandwiched between strangers, I remember six words from that class: "Child's Pose is always an option." Each time the instructor said it, I dropped into it like a dead fly and felt immediate relief. Ease rushed through my body. It felt amazing! But then I'd look up and see everyone holding Downward-Facing Dog. *How? How is everyone holding this torturous pose for so long?* I wouldn't have believed it was even possible if I hadn't seen it with my own eyes.

My thoughts changed: *Okay, yoga people aren't weird. They are crazy and like to torture themselves.* I struggled to hold Downward-Facing Dog because I was convinced I needed to be as strong as everyone else, but it physically hurt. I had zero upper body strength. Each time I surrendered to Child's Pose, my breath and heart rate slowed down, and I felt so good.

Then the teacher turned off the lights. We lay still in Savasana, the final resting pose, and I disappeared into another reality. It was glorious.

I walked out of that studio and felt the warm evening air on my skin. The full moon and white stucco wall had more texture than before. "Wow, I feel high," I told my friend, and we started laughing. "Also, I feel like jello. This is cool."

I share this story for every person who steps out of their comfort zone to take any group class. The beauty of a group class is that it can be motivating. If you stick with it, it can help you grow stronger. The downside is that it's often competitive, which makes it easy to override the wisdom of your body and hurt yourself. In this first yoga class, my body knew it needed to rest in Child's Pose. It knew that I didn't have the physical strength to keep up with the level of athleticism in the room. My body didn't care what anyone else was doing. My body wasn't comparing itself. My body was doing what it needed to do. Over the years, most group classes compelled me to override my body's signals and push myself beyond my strength and flexibility. As a consequence, I hurt myself a lot. If you're starting out in a group class, listen to your body; it knows what you are capable of, and it doesn't care what anyone else is doing. This will save you unnecessary harm that will ultimately keep you from enjoying your fitness journey.

I'm not saying that once you realize you're competing with others you'll naturally listen to the wisdom of the body. This is a major healing puzzle piece because it takes time to undo the overriding that happens, especially in group classes. It helps if the instructor reminds you that it isn't a competition, but you still have to learn how to listen to your body. If you're reading this and wondering, *What is wisdom of the body? How do I learn to listen to my body? How do I stop overriding my body's signals?* Feel free to skip ahead to chapter 4: step 2. It will teach you how to identify the pain you're living with and open a dialogue with the wisdom of your body.

I spent many years developing a conversation with my body. Once a week, I stopped rushing around, being led by my thoughts, and took a few minutes to listen and write about it. It was hard. Most of the time I wrote how cold I was because it was snowing, and I wasn't used to the snow. I struggled to believe that my body was intelligent. I grew up learning, "Mind over matter. If you don't mind, it don't matter." But one injury at a time, I have learned to listen deeper, which has taught me how to feel what was happening in my body. I learned the difference between pain from weakness, pain from old injuries, pain from a pinched nerve or muscle spasm, pain from stress, and pain from overuse. By listening to your body, you too will learn from its wisdom.

CHAPTER 1: CONCUSSION

One piece of healing is recognizing when you're adding stress to your pain by pushing through it. Stop moving so much. Take the time to be still, to feel your body, to ask it what it needs, and to listen to its response. At first, it may be a whisper. The conversation may be superficial. You may only feel the temperature of your skin or the aches and pains, but with practice, you and your body can develop a powerful open conversation. So powerful, in fact, that when a doctor or someone in a place of authority tells you what your body needs or how long it will take for your body to heal, you'll be able to check in with your highest authority, the wisdom of your body, and decide if that's true for you, or if you need to find a new practitioner to work with on your healing journey.

If you want to speed up the conversation with your body's intelligence, ask yourself:

1. *Does this step on the healing path feel safe to me?* ❏ Yes ❏ No
2. *Is this an empowering step?* ❏ Yes ❏ No
3. *Am I gaining wisdom and feeling more freedom within?* ❏ Yes ❏ No

If the answer to any of these questions is "No!" then it isn't a healing step that's grounded in loving kindness, which is the first step to healing head and neck pain. I will go over this more in chapter 4 and 5.

Here's another story that shows these questions in action. I went to a hot yoga class, which is the equivalent of practicing yoga in a sauna with a bunch of other sweaty bodies. I had never met the male yoga instructor and had no idea what to expect. He didn't know me or how long I'd been practicing yoga. Heck, he didn't even know my name. All he knew was that I was a new, young, attractive female in his hot yoga class.

Halfway through class, we were all in a standing balance pose. We began reaching toward our extended foot. I latched two of my fingers around my big toe and extended it out to the side. This was a rare moment for me. It had taken years of practice to reach my toes. I felt so much joy as I extended the leg open, I was basking in the newness of the pose. I took a breath and held myself steady.

Imagine the shock when this very buff and sweaty instructor stepped right between my legs, as close to me as he could, grabbed under the heel of my foot that was out to my side and pulled it even further out. I could see the sweat on his neck and chest. He was inches from my face. Then he let go, and I fell off balance trying to catch my breath. After class, I was very confused. I am a yoga instructor and a massage therapist who enjoys deep adjustments, so why did I feel violated?

I had to ask myself these questions:

Does this step on the healing path feel safe to me? No. "No" is a complete answer, but in case you're wondering why, here's why: He could have pulled one of my muscles. His adjustment felt sexual. Invasive. He didn't even witness my practice for one full class before coming in for a very personal adjustment.

Is this an empowering step? No, because I'm trying to justify his action and make what he did feel okay when I don't feel okay. I spent the rest of class feeling anxiety because I wanted to run out of the room, but didn't want to be dramatic.

Am I gaining wisdom and feeling more freedom within? No. In his class, he could do whatever he wanted, and I didn't have a say. That wasn't okay with me, so I never went back.

CHAPTER 1: CONCUSSION

Instead, I found instructors who respected my space, offered clear and appropriate adjustments, and taught in a way that made me feel safe.

JACUZZI CONCUSSION

When I was 12 years old, my cousins and I were playing in an empty jacuzzi. They were hiding inside of the tub under the leather cover. I thought it would be funny to trap them inside, so I climbed on top of it. Then they started kicking hard. At first, I tried to imagine I was in an ocean fighting waves because they were taking turns kicking me back and forth. Then they started kicking together, and I yelled "Calm down, you guys. Stop!" I could see myself being whipped off the edge, and I panicked. I had to get off, but it was all I could do to hold on as they laughed and kicked harder. Eventually, they got tired, and I slid off one side, feeling dizzy and angry. The second my feet hit the ground, I ran to tell my grandma and get them in trouble.

The next moment, my slippery socks glided over the slick floor, my feet flew out from under me, my body suspended in midair, and the back of my head slammed into the side of the jacuzzi. Just like in the cartoons, I saw black and then stars. I crawled up the stairs on all fours, the world shifting from black to sparkles, black to twinkling, black to normal. My head was pulsing and throbbing. I was completely disoriented. When I entered the living room upstairs, still on all fours, the colors in the room were dim, then bright. I tried to ignore the throbbing in my head, the dizziness, the low-level headache. But by the time I got home hours later, the symptoms still hadn't lessened.

My parents rushed me to Urgent Care, and the doctor informed them I had a concussion. I was told to rest, take Tylenol, and that I would be back to normal in three weeks. Unfortunately, it took much longer.

After this injury, I grew accustomed to living with head and neck pain that came and went without warning. Pain became an unwanted companion I could not shake. I had two approaches to dealing with it: complaining about it or pushing through and ignoring it. I didn't have any tools to turn to for relief. One I wish I had known about earlier is CranioSacral therapy.

HEALING PUZZLE PIECE
#2 - CranioSacral Therapy

CranioSacral therapy helped me recover from the chronic head and neck pain that came from multiple concussions. My first experience receiving CranioSacral therapy was surprising. The woman working with me said to take off my shoes and climb onto the table. I had received many massages and was ready to undress and get under the sheets. I can't remember if I had uncomfortable clothes on, but a note to those interested in trying this out: wear comfortable clothes.

I got myself situated, and the extra foam cushion on her table was heavenly. She placed her hands under the heels of my feet, and I felt my entire body stiffen up. Nobody had ever held my feet for such a long time. At first I thought, *This is weird*. After a few more minutes, however, my body began to melt. I felt myself drifting between relaxation and sleep. She placed my feet on the table and moved her hands to the top of my ankles. My muscles let go even more. A few minutes later, she placed her hands over my thighs and then onto my lower and upper ribs. I felt my body tighten again. She didn't stay there as long. Then she put her hands under the base of my head, and I felt my eyes start to water. I drifted off into a restful sleep. I'm not sure how long she was there.

I woke up when she ended the session by placing one hand under my head and one hand under my sacrum, which is the triangular bone at the base of the spine just beneath the lower back. She held this position for close to fifteen minutes. It felt like I was floating in water. I had to open my eyes multiple times because I felt dizzy from the sensation of rocking. My eyes started to water again. At first, I fought the urge to cry, but eventually I let go. She gave me a tissue and held her hands there longer. I asked her why it felt like I was floating and why I could no longer feel her hands. She explained how CranioSacral helps the nervous system relax by releasing restricted connective tissues, blood flow, and cerebral spinal fluids. At the time, all I understood was that she had somehow gotten the fluid systems in my body to circulate better. I didn't know how she loosened the connective tissues or what the connective tissues were, but I knew I felt amazing. So I went back.

After a few sessions, I noticed that every time she had her fingers under the base of my skull, I felt immediate relief. I asked her to explain it to me again. This time she explained that her hands were holding my occipital bone. This is the bone that took the impact when I fell on the jacuzzi. It's the bone at the base of the skull where the spinal cord and nerves pass through.

When this bone got pressed up, the muscles around it tightened. No amount of manual adjustments from massage therapists or chiropractors could get rid of the pain for more than a couple of weeks. This restriction in the occipital bone created pain in my muscles and nerves for years.

What are nerves?
Nerves are similar to electrical circuits. They carry messages between the brain and the body.

Why do nerves matter?

Think about everything you are doing right now. Your eyes have to move from side to side to read. Your hands, arms, and eyes help you text, drive, etc. Your brain is communicating with your body via nerves. It is telling them what you need to do to absorb the information in this book, to not text the wrong person, to drive safely, and so on. Your nerves and nervous system take in information and figure out appropriate ways to respond. The nerves matter because they are in constant dialogue with your central nervous system. The nerves tell the brain what needs to be done. The brain tells the muscles what to do, and the muscles tell the bones what to do.

Where are the nerves located?

At the base of the skull there is a circular hole called the foramen magnum, where the spinal cord and 12 cranial nerves travel through to communicate back and forth with the brain.

The occipital bone at the base of the skull sits directly above the first cervical vertebrae, which is the beginning of the spine. This area tends to get over-compressed because of modern living (working on computers, looking at cell phones, and sitting with a forward head position). When also compressed from an injury, it restricts healthy blood and nerve flow. In my case, my poor posture due to weak muscles and pain from injury resulted in a consistent pressure at the base of my skull that always returned.

One solution is to become aware of the circular hole at the base of the skull and to notice the range of motion in your neck. *Is there limiting space in the neck where the nerves flow? Do you have forward head posture? Do you look down excessively? Or do you have a combination of the two?* If so, work on lifting your gaze, pressing the head back, increasing the range of motion in the neck and allow more space in the neck for the nerves to flow with ease.

CHAPTER 1: CONCUSSION

The three photos below show the hole at the base of the occipital bone, the foramen magnum, and where the spinal cord and nerves pass through.

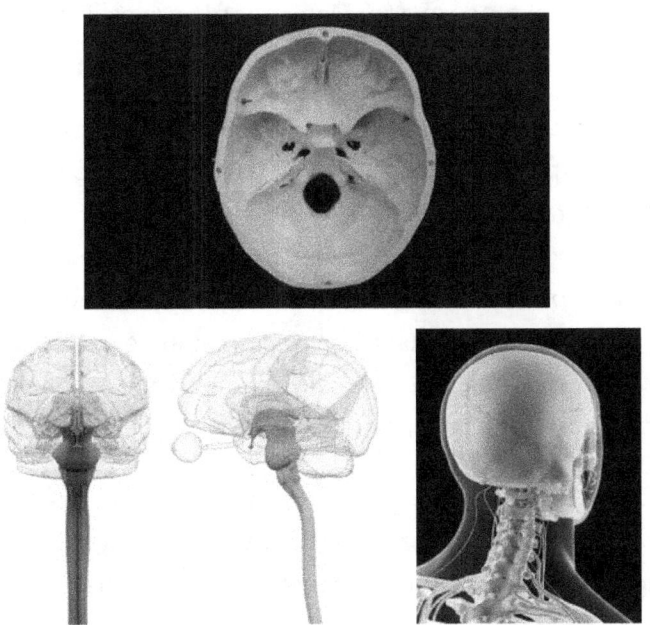

Before this CranioSacral session, the nerves in my neck were impinged and inflamed, which caused a recurring sharp pain in my head and neck. The muscles in my neck chronically pulled and tightened to protect the hurt area, long after the injury. This tension restricted blood flow, and the cerebral spinal fluid from flowing freely throughout my body. Produced in the brain, Cerebrospinal fluid is there to provide protection, nourishment, and waste removal. Ideally, this fluid circulates without restriction.

After this CranioSacral session, the restriction at the base of my skull was completely released. The chronic neck pain I'd been living with for years was gone—and it never returned! The cerebral spinal fluid was able to flow without restriction and that continued to be true long after this CranioSacral session.

I share this story because many live with tension in this area of the body, some who have suffered from previous head or neck injuries, some who are impacted by the poor posture that comes from living in this technological modern age. Many people are calling this condition "Tech Neck."

The simple understanding of this important part of your anatomy--where the occiput, spinal cord, and nerves are working hard to transfer information through the entire body--can help you immediately. If you'd like an exercise to help create space in this area, skip ahead to chapter 7 and practice the first exercise in the neck section. It can also help to lay with your occipital bone resting at the edge of a foam roller or at the edge of a bed. Then visualize the occipital bone relaxing and feel space around the foramen magnum.

Another thing to consider is when you experience impact from falling hard on your tailbone. Anyone who has had this experience knows how it can knock the wind out of you and that's because your nerves are affected.

What happens to the nerves when you slam your sacrum?

The triangular bone at the base of the spine that ends with the tailbone is the sacrum. When it is jolted with force, the impact runs up the spine fast, and the nerves and muscles respond to the pain. They most likely contract. In some cases they continue to contract, spasm, or create unnecessary pain until they've had massage, CranioSacral therapy, and corrective movement. Falling on your tailbone and misaligning your sacrum can cause pain in the upper body. It can also bruise your tailbone, causing pain in the low back and hips. Think of the sacrum, the spine, the spinal cord, the brain, and the bones around the brain all as one unit. When any part of that unit is hurt, it is felt through the entire central nervous system.

CHAPTER 1: CONCUSSION

CranioSacral therapy releases stored pain in the body that massage and other manual therapies may not be able to address. When stored tension in one part of the body releases, it can often be felt in other parts of the body. For example, if you grind your teeth or tighten your jaw when stressed, or if you've had a lot of dental work, your jaw pain may be causing or adding to your head and neck pain. CranioSacral therapy can release jaw tension and relieve some, if not all, head and neck pain.

CHAPTER 2

WHIPLASH

Whiplash is a common injury. One of the most well-known whiplash injuries happens when you are rear-ended in a car accident. If the headrest is not directly behind your head to brace the impact, then the force causes the head to extend all the way back, over the headrest, beyond the normal range of motion. This is called hyper extension of the neck. Another common way people experience whiplash is on roller coasters and water slides. Whiplash can also happen from slipping, playing sports, skiing, getting into a fight or in other ways.

Hyperextension happens when the muscles, tendons, and ligaments in the neck stretch backward beyond a normal range of motion. The muscles in your neck are meant to stretch into extension. The tendons are in place to connect the muscles to the bones. Muscles move the bones, tendons secure the attachment of muscles to bones, and ligaments connect bone to bone. More dense than muscles and tendons, the ligaments are designed to keep joints from over stretching. When your muscles, tendons, and ligaments overstretch, it leads to instability and weakness in the neck. It's very common for other muscles to then overwork to try and stabilize the injured area. This is how you get muscles that are excessively tight, combined with muscles that are excessively weak. To make matters worse, sometimes in whiplash the head swings in both directions, moving forward into hyper flexion as well, which is when the head forcefully drops toward the chest.

This forceful motion of the head whipping backward and forward stresses the muscles, tendons, ligaments, and nerves in the neck in both directions. Pain is not always felt right away and in severe cases, pain doesn't go away on its own.

What happens to the nerves when you experience whiplash?
Whiplash can damage the nerves, stress out the neck muscles, and affect communication between the brain and the body. The good news is that nerves are doing their best to recover, as the body is always doing what it can to optimize your well-being. If dull or sharp pain persists from damage in the area, it needs treatment, such as movement, CranioSacral therapy, and massage, so the central nervous system can function without added stress. If pain persists, see a primary care doctor who can set you up with an MRI and give you a referral to a trusted doctor of physical therapy or chiropractic care. Insurance should cover the majority of costs, and professionals with years of study are ideally the first ones to work with your severe injury. Many doctors have massage therapists or personal trainers on staff to whom you can transition after your initial sessions.

The nervous system is complex, and when you experience a traumatic or unexpected injury the body remembers. The body's response to injury is to tighten, protect, and send in scar tissue, blood, and whatever else is needed to help the hurt area. Once the acute pain has lessened, it needs stabilizing and strengthening movement as well as massage to get the body back to functioning without pain.

CHAPTER 2: WHIPLASH

Here are a few stories about the unfortunate ways I got whiplash and didn't know it. Maybe you'll realize you had whiplash too and weren't aware of it. At the end of each story, you'll find another healing puzzle piece.

AMUSEMENT PARK WHIPLASH

When I was 10-years-old, weaving through the long line to the Indiana Jones ride at Disneyland with my family, I remember the warning signs. They basically said, "Due to the jerky motion of this ride, whiplash is a possibility and for those who've experienced whiplash, they are likely to have it happen again." I stepped into the rollercoaster, which was designed as a jeep with no head or neck support. The ride started. The jeep jerked forward, and the muscles in my neck fought to hold my head upright. The constant stopping and starting and quick turns were a lot to handle, but I felt okay.

Then a gigantic concrete looking wrecking ball rolled toward the jeep as we sped toward it. At the last second, the jeep took a sudden drop to dodge the ball; the roller coaster jerked down, and my head whipped backward. I saw black, or maybe it was the ride. Then my neck felt numb, and I was afraid to turn my head.

As the day went on, my neck got increasingly achy and sore, but I kept going on rides. I was a kid who complained a lot, so my parents didn't take my whining seriously. I learned to live with a stiff neck and forgot about this moment, until almost two decades later.

In my late twenties, after I'd recovered from many head and neck injuries, I went to a water park. I had forgotten how painful whiplash was and that it could happen on a ride. Full of excitement, I sat in the inner tube, ready to plunge down the steep water slide. The woman working at the top gave my tube an extra push down. As it rushed up a steep wall of water, I was giddy. Then my head flung so far back I could see the lady at the top of the slide waiting to push the next person down. My neck jerked back up, and I saw my belly button. I reached back and held my head in place until the ride was over. The rest of the day was spent watching my family enjoy the rides.

I wanted to go on the scariest ride and considered it, but I couldn't ignore the dull ache in my neck. So instead, I watched as groups of 3-6 people sat in a large inner tube and spiraled down a wide slide into a circular area that resembled a gigantic toilet bowl. There were waves pushing them forcefully back and forth. Each time the inner tube hit one of the waves, their bodies bounced up, and they grabbed tight onto the handle bars. The screams and laughter made me want to go on the ride even more.

But, in the 20 to 30 minutes I stood watching, I counted around 6 people who experienced whiplash from the ride. When their inner tube hit the waves, their bodies bounced up and their heads whipped backward into full hyper extension. I was grateful I had the awareness to not hurt myself more by going on the ride, like I'd done as a child, even if it meant missing out on a few fun moments.

If you have experienced whiplash or have chronic head and neck pain, you may need to sit out some of the rides. Mainly, the ones that don't have head and neck support. Ask yourself if the short-lived fun will be worth it if it increases your head and neck pain or brings back old pain. If it feels worth it, go for it, but if your neck takes a hit, like mine did, don't go on any more rides. It's definitely not worth it. Instead, be proactive with your choices. Choose the option that's best for your body. This will help you recover faster and keep your neck muscles, tendons, and ligaments more stable.

CHAPTER 2: WHIPLASH

HEALING PUZZLE PIECE
#3 - Yoga Therapy

I practiced yoga for many years before I found yoga therapy, but from day one I found comfort and healing from resting into Child's Pose. Before I get into the details of Yoga therapy, I want to share this pose with you. These two photos show two variations of Child's Pose. The one with props is more restorative and accessible to most bodies. For others, Child's Pose with no props will feel great. Both poses help relieve nausea, relax your nervous system, and create a sense of safety in your body and mind. Start practicing one or both of these today and notice how it helps reduce head and neck pain. Then check out yoga therapy or restorative yoga options in your area or skip ahead to chapter 7 to begin to build on your self-practice.

There are many forms of yoga therapy nowadays, and each has a unique approach. I was fortunate enough to study under two instructors who came from different yoga therapy backgrounds: the ViniYoga tradition and the Structural Yoga lineage. When it came time to choose an instructor to mentor me during the 300 hour yoga teacher training at YogaWorks, I decided to work with Lakshmi, the *Structural Yoga Therapy* instructor. In the weeks prior to choosing an instructor, I took both classes and observed how I felt during and after. Although I felt better mentally after Vini Yoga classes, I often left with new aches and pains. In contrast, when I took *Structural Yoga Therapy* with Lakshmi, I left feeling as though she had a magic wand that vanished the pain I was experiencing.

In many classes, Lakshmi focused on teaching 22 postures from the joint freeing series. She learned from Mukunda Styles, a physical therapist, dedicated yoga practitioner, author of *Structural Yoga Therapy*, and the man who created the joint freeing series. He bridged the two worlds in a brilliant way that makes it accessible to every-body. This series taught me that I have many hyper mobile joints, meaning I can move my joints beyond a healthy range of motion. This can be true for anybody, in some or many joints. More commonly, the joints are stiff and lack range of motion. The joint freeing series helps bring mobility to stiff joints and strength to hyper mobile joints. This series gave me the stability I needed to finally perform a proper push up. It was also the initial foundation I needed to heal my head and neck pain before moving forward with more strength training.

Strength was something I had been working hard at building in yoga classes for years, but, because of my injuries and hyper mobile joints, I kept hurting myself. The repetitive sun salutations and standing poses typically found in a yoga flow class--plank, upward dog, downward dog, Warrior poses, forward folds, and standing up quickly, in sequence--kept aggravating my shoulder weakness and hip instability. I used to think the weakness was in my mind, that one day I'd get stronger. While I did end up getting stronger, it wasn't from repeating the exercises that were continuing to aggravate my injuries; it was from letting go of the Yoga Flow classes and instead practicing Yoga Therapy.

Yoga therapy is the gift that keeps on giving. It teaches you how to slow down, be present, and take the time to unwind years of stress, pain, and trauma. Most of the westernized world has been taught to push through pain, to challenge the body with exercise, to abuse the body, or not care about it at all. Yoga therapy helps you unlearn all of this and relearn how to be still and surrender to the present moment. Healing happens in the stillness and slow movements. If you think you'd benefit from the joint freeing series, get the book, *Structural Yoga Therapy* and dive in. For more yoga therapy resources, flip to the movement resources in chapter 12.

CHAPTER 2: WHIPLASH

CAR ACCIDENT WHIPLASH

When I was 15, I was sitting in the middle of the back seat of a jeep, hot air blowing in through the windows. I was holding onto my friend's legs, one on each side, because I didn't have a seat belt on, and the kid driving was swerving through the desert. He raced along the edge of steep sand dunes.

The next moment, a holographic image of my dead mother's face appeared through the window. I turned to tell my friend, and the jeep fishtailed. My head whipped back and forward as the jeep tipped over the edge of the sand dune. For a second, we seemed to balance on two wheels. And then there were legs and arms crashing into me as the car suspended in the air before landing on the roof. I don't remember the impact. I'm pretty sure my head hit the roof. Everything went black. Then I heard a voice say, *Get out of the car.* I crawled out one of the windows.

All I could think about was how much trouble I was going to get into for getting into the car of a boy I didn't know. One of my friends had a purple bruise over her collarbone; it looked like a golf ball was lodged under her skin. The three of us decided to get away from the car, away from the boys, away from any evidence we were there at all. We jumped into the back of a truck of Mexican workers, then hitched a ride back to school where two of us hid out in the bathroom. We convinced our friend with the broken collar bone to get help from the school nurse and to not rat us out.

In the bathroom, the other girl showed me her back and the seatbelt burned across her skin. Our adrenaline was high. I remember finding friends in the cafeteria and telling them what happened. They said we were stupid to hide and we needed to go get checked out by the nurse. I kept telling myself I was fine, even though my neck and right shoulder were in excruciating pain, and I had a headache. I figured if I wasn't hurt maybe I wouldn't get in as much trouble. We went to the nurse, and she called our parents.

My parents took me to urgent care. I had whiplash, a concussion, and I don't remember what they said about my shoulder. All I know is the right side of my neck and shoulder never healed right. Most likely that's because a few days after the car accident I tried to run through the pain during a track and field practice. I got a stabbing pain in my upper right shoulder and found it hard to breathe. This pain stuck with me for over a decade. It returned every time I ran. This may sound repetitive, but it bears repeating: give your body time to heal after an injury. I learned this the hard way.

HEALING PUZZLE PIECE
#4 - Chiropractic Care

I remember the first time a chiropractor held my head: I was 10-years-old and terrified. My armpits were sweaty, my eyes watered, and I had the urge to run away. Maybe I'd seen too many movies where a guy twists someone's neck and kills the person. I told myself, *it's okay. I'll be okay.* Eventually the chiropractor twisted my head to the side and then forcefully took it a little further. My whole neck made a popping sound, and then he adjusted the other side. Next, he had me lay face down and pressed on my middle back. More popping traveled up my back. I loved that part; I still do.

When the adjustments were over, I experienced relief in my head and neck for a while, but the pain returned and that chiropractor never helped me understand why. Over the years, I've received chiropractic adjustments from 10 different chiropractors in three states, and I can tell you that each of them approached spinal adjustments in their own way. This is to say that there is not one chiropractic approach. Some helped me for a short period of time; some made lasting changes. This is true for all healing professionals.

After a handful of male chiropractors who cranked on my neck with no lasting results, I went to Anne Fang when I was in my mid 20s. She taught me that my scalene neck muscles, on the right side, were contracting and pulling up on my top two ribs. The scalene muscle was pulling my ribs out of alignment and affecting my neck. Before this moment, I had no idea my upper ribs were contributing to my neck pain. After seeing her for half a year, my life was forever changed for the better. She massaged the scalene muscles before and after each adjustment. She also cracked my neck and put it back when it was out of alignment, but her technique was focused on adjusting my top two vertebrae, not the entire neck. When I think back, I don't have a clue what the earlier chiropractors did with my neck. What was out? What did they put back in? Why did it feel good right after only to have the same pain return? These are questions Anne Fang answered. She created lasting change, not just maintenance.

Another chiropractor at The Movement Chiropractic in Maple Grove, Minnesota helped me regain extension in my neck in my early 30s. I had done so much work on my neck that I figured it was as good as it would get. I was grateful I could look over my shoulders without pain, and it had been years since I'd pinched a nerve in my neck. So maybe I couldn't look at the wall behind me, there are worse things. I went to work as a massage therapist for this chiropractor, and he took an x-ray of my neck. He showed me where my neck vertebrae were straight and needed to have a c-curve. He said if I saw him for a few months regularly, he could restore the natural curve in the cervical vertebrae. What was new to me with this chiropractor was that he incorporated stretching, strengthening, and massage into his practice.

After a few months, I was able to look at the wall behind me with no pain. This was a miraculous healing puzzle piece! The combination of movement and massage with chiropractic care is the best form of chiropractic care I've come across. Many chiropractors work with massage therapists because they know, if they don't change the soft tissues and work out scar tissue, the muscles will continue to pull on the spine. Many more chiropractors are beginning to incorporate movement into their practices too.

I recommend searching the Foundation Training website to see if there is a chiropractor with this training nearby because that means they are likely incorporating movement into their practice. Foundation Training is an incredible resource that gives you the ability to change the way you move and correct any physical imbalances you're living with. To learn more about Foundation Training, flip to the movement resources in chapter 12.

CHAPTER 3

DEPRESSION

Depression is an internal and often unseen injury that doesn't always show up right after a head injury. It isn't always diagnosed, and even when it is diagnosed, it isn't always recognized as a side effect of traumatic brain injury. Many studies show the connection between mild-traumatic brain injuries and depression. Cognitive FX is one of the best sites I've found to discuss the effects of concussions. Their article, "Depression After a Concussion: Why You Feel This Way and How to Start Healing," breaks down the behavioral activation system in our brains:

> "You can think of the behavioral activation system as our brain's default setting. It makes us curious and eager to learn. It helps us feel rewarded for mastering a topic or experiencing something pleasurable. It's an important part of why we engage with the world and the people around us. But in the background, the behavioral inhibition system is monitoring everything we do. It's watching out for loss, and it tells us whenever we've experienced a loss. And

if we experience what it believes are too many losses, it pulls back on the reins, dampening (or completely disrupting) the behavioral activation system." (https://www.cognitivefxusa.com/blog/depression-after-concussion-and-post-concussion-syndrome)

Anyone who has had a minor-traumatic traumatic brain injury knows how it feels to no longer feel the way they once did. You have to deal with not only the physical effects, but also the mental side effects. However, many of us are unprepared for the mood swings, the crying spells, the dizziness, the lack of motivation to be around peers, the isolation, the frustration with our bodies and minds, and the feeling that something is wrong with us. The description above articulates what I struggled with for a decade: my behavioral inhibition system got triggered too much and became highly aware of the many losses I was sustaining. It took over. I became cautious, fearful, indecisive, and anxious. I spent a decade searching for ways to ignite curiosity and motivation, for ways to be proactive. At the time, I didn't know this was my way of reigniting the basic behavioral activation system.

For anyone struggling with this, "Depression After a Concussion: Why You Feel This Way and How to Start Healing" says it best:

> "It's so important to understand: There isn't something wrong with you for feeling this way. Your brain – specifically, your behavioral inhibition system – is just trying to protect you from further loss, and it's messing with your feelings in the process."

I know a woman who was hit by a truck in her late 20s when serving in the Peace Corps. She was left for dead on the side of the road in Guatemala after suffering a traumatic head injury. When she returned home in a wheelchair with limited mobility, she had to work to get back to her normal functions. Once she was up and moving again, the mental struggle began. She battled suicidal thoughts. Family and friends watched out for her for over a year before she was diagnosed with depression and given the proper medication that allowed her brain to function in a way that allowed her to move forward. Now she's living the life she always dreamed of with a husband "and two children in Wyoming.

I too have struggled with depression and mood swings since my first concussion in 8th grade. But the loneliness, worthlessness, and sorrow increased after my second concussion. In my youth, I used drugs to escape the pain, both recreational and medical. I was reckless with my body. I took what was presented to me--pain pills, ecstasy, Adderall, and psychedelics. Thankfully, I never took the wrong combination. My sister likes to remind me that I tried to overdose on Pepto Bismol once. It seems funny now, but at the time I felt like my brain was covered in darkness, and I was searching for an easy way out. I figured downing a bottle of Pepto Bismol would be the easiest way to drift into an endless sleep.

In college, after my third and most traumatic concussion, my depression and mood swings worsened. I was taking meditation classes at Naropa University, where we'd sit in a circle on the floor, take a moment to sit upright and bow together, and then check-in by speaking from our hearts. I left each class feeling exhausted and sad. I cried a lot; I'd break into uncontrollable sobs multiple times a week, sometimes daily.

I felt helpless, hopeless, and tired all the time. I thought it was a side effect of having an open heart and told myself I had to learn to live with the sadness. It never occurred to me that my most recent head injury was affecting my mental health. I was down on myself for feeling tired, for being sad, and for having time to feel horrible. I learned to live with the depressing feelings, and they became a huge part of me.

When I was 32, a decade after my traumatic brain injury, my depression reached a climax. I had moved seven times in one year, from one state or city to the next. Sometimes I only lived in one place for two weeks before realizing it was not where I "needed" to be. I told myself that I liked adventures and that's why I was moving so much. I tried to embrace loneliness, but the truth was that when I wasn't reinventing myself and re-building my life from scratch, I was depressed. I needed to live on the edge to feel anything other than the returning sadness and hopelessness.

At the end of all the moving, I fell into an emotionally abusive relationship and told myself it was love, but deep down I knew it wasn't. That's when I thought I might lose my mind. I felt like I was having a mental breakdown. I remember walking around a park on a beautiful sunny day, and I couldn't find an ounce of joy inside. I walked to the beach and felt empty. The beach had always been my happy place, the one place that could lift the burdens and whisper sweet reminders of happiness—but not anymore. My mind raced at a speed I couldn't calm. I had visions of becoming a person who lives out of her car, talks to herself, and doesn't trust anyone. I felt as though I was a few decisions away from losing my grip on reality. I share this as a reminder to anyone living with a traumatic brain injury or for anyone who knows someone who's experienced a TBI. It can take years for depression to reach a peak. Be gentle with yourself. Be kind to your loved ones and encourage them to seek help if you notice them spiraling into depression.

It was a blessing that I knew I had to ask for help. I knew the amount of mental struggle I was living with was unbearable. I didn't want to become a homeless drug addict, which seemed like the next best option to suicide. I refused to become a suicide statistic. I knew it was time to change the depressive programming in my brain. I started searching for ways to heal the brain, and this is what I found:

CHAPTER 3: DEPRESSION

HEALING PUZZLE PIECES #5
Vision Board Creation, Cognitive Behavioral Therapy, & Removing Amalgam Fillings

The puzzle pieces that helped heal my head traumas and depression were presented into my life over two decades. When I was in high school feeling depressed after my jeep accident and second concussion, I came across *You Can Heal Your Life* by Louise Hay and *The Power of Now* by Eckhart Tolle. I learned about the power of positive affirmations and I posted them all over my room, so I could transform my negative thoughts into positive ones. I imagined myself living in Colorado, going to college, getting a degree, and eventually becoming a writer and yoga teacher.

I moved to Colorado when I was 19. I went to Naropa University, enrolled in writing and yoga classes, and placed the same positive affirmations all over my room. It was harder to stay positive in Colorado because I didn't know anyone. I missed my family. Colorado was a complete culture shock from being raised in Las Vegas, NV. On top of that, learning how to meditate just highlighted the pain in my body and mind. I did my best to focus on being grateful and positive, even when I felt exhausted and sad.

After a year and a half, I'd grown used to Colorado. The weather changes, the cultural shifts, and the constant reminders from the Buddhist University to live from an open heart. I made new friends. I fell in love. I started listening to my body's intelligence and learning about the healing power of yoga. Then I experienced my most traumatic head injury. After this injury, I hated my body. I felt trapped in darkness. I cried all the time. I slept for ten to twelve hours a day, and all I wanted to do was sleep more.

After a few months of feeling this way, I made my first vision board. One of the most powerful images I found was of an Asian woman resting on a massage table with two hands under her skull. I loved that image. I saw peace in her face and gentleness in the hands holding her; the image made me feel better. I stared at it a lot when I wasn't having crying fits. I'd imagine myself in her position and myself as the healing practitioner. I wanted to be as close to that image as possible.

A couple of years later when I was experiencing severe head and neck pain and sharing this with a yoga student, she gave me the number of a CranioSacral therapist. I went to see the therapist and was shocked to find that she held my head the same way as the woman in the vision board photo. This helped heal my head and neck pain, and it guided me to become a massage and CranioSacral therapist. This work gave me clients who helped support me financially, and one of those clients was a woman who looked almost identical to the one from my vision board. We worked together three times a week for years, and I experienced all the peace, healing, and gentleness I'd envisioned. It was surreal.

At the same time, I was given the book *Waking the Tiger* by Dr. Peter A. Levin, and it discussed Somatic Experiencing, a body-oriented healing approach. It described what happens in our body when we experience trauma and ways to heal it. I searched for a therapist certified in Somatic Experiencing. Since I was a massage therapist, I found this work intriguing. The sessions I received helped me feel safe in my body by giving me resources to feel the objects around me and stay present when traumatic emotions arose. I learned to track my emotions, something I hadn't had the ability to do previously. This showed me how to actively relax and rest into a parasympathetic state. After a handful of sessions, I thought I was healed. I soon moved away from the area and stopped working with her.

CHAPTER 3: DEPRESSION

Then, after moving seven times in one year, I was at the peak of my depression. I returned to what had helped me: I created a vision board. I made a collage with smiling faces, and even though I couldn't see joy in the moment, the images gave me a glimmer of hope for the future. Instead of crying at night with no purpose, I began writing and performing poetry to cope with the emotions and the emptiness I felt. I forced myself to wake up early, go on walks, work out, eat right, write, and serve people in the healing arts. I told myself I would get better and one day I would enjoy life again.

Then I met a man straight off my vision board! He had the same smile and facial hair from the photo I'd been staring at for months. It was kind of creepy when he came into my room the first time. He stood beside the vision board and said, "That's me."

"I know. It's crazy!" I said. It's a good thing he didn't think I was a stalker.

With this new man in my life, the future seemed promising, but I was still down and out. I was dating someone kind, sweet-hearted, loving, committed, dedicated, adventurous, yet I could barely smile. It was made even more obvious because every time I saw him, his smile lit up the room. I needed to become the happy person I saw on the vision board, yet there I was having crying spells—often. I was embarrassed because it was out of my control. I knew I couldn't keep living with depression, so I went down a Google rabbit hole and emerged with evidence that Cognitive Behavioral Therapy can help the brain recover from traumatic brain injuries. This was a major healing puzzle piece!

I'd never heard of Cognitive Behavioral Therapy, but I decided to give it a try with someone who used scientific evidence based meditation skills and art therapy. Fortunately, my insurance covered it, giving me the freedom to go weekly. We worked together for almost a year, during which I continued to eat well and exercise daily, even if it was just a short walk. I realized that I had major gut issues. From nutritionist friends, I knew that the gut is our second brain and that it needs to be healthy in order for the body and mind to be healthy. I discovered that Acupuncture was also covered under my insurance, so I started seeing someone who traded me herbs in exchange for massages. After a few months, my stomach started to feel better, but the depression lingered. The crying spells went away, but the heavy darkness hung around.

I had heard repeatedly that amalgam fillings leak mercury after a few years and can cause depression. For years, I'd told myself it was just another way people were trying to get more money, but a few things made me reconsider: 1. I could taste metal in my mouth all the time. 2. The dentist showed me five fillings that were beginning to crack, where the mercury was leaking, and said if I didn't have them refilled soon, I'd need crowns. I signed up for dental insurance to offset the cost and spent thousands of dollars to get all 10 taken out. I'd had the same amalgam fillings since I was 10, so, 20+ years later, it was high time to get rid of them.

A few weeks after they were removed, I felt a drastic change! I remember walking down the street after it rained and the sun was shining on a leaf that had a drop of water on it. I stood there in the sunshine, witnessing the reflecting light bouncing off that drip of water, and I felt a soft breeze on my face. I smelled the fresh rain. I saw the emerald green of the leaves and had a sense it was all going to get better. I missed being immersed in the moment, with no black curtain blocking me from the beauty of the present.

This moment spurred me to integrate more self-care practices: I started taking DHA/EPA oils to help my brain; I drank warm lemon water with apple cider vinegar every morning to help cleanse my liver, and I took CBD occasionally when I experienced overwhelming emotions, which happened far less often. The CBD helped me relax and remember to slow down, and not fear the depression returning. I included myself in the prayer for all human beings to be happy and free. I stayed in therapy every other week for a year to stay focused on rebuilding my life, my career, and most importantly, my inner joy. After all of this—I felt better.

I share this not to overwhelm you with all the things you have to do, but to illustrate that healing is not a linear or immediate path. It's a puzzle, and the pieces in this book are here as options to help you fill in the parts of your healing puzzle. No matter what, remember: there is no shame in asking for help. It's okay to cry and feel the whole range of emotions. It's okay to feel nothing. It's okay to feel too much and to admit you're depressed, to take medicine if you need it, to find your unique path through the rugged and crappy terrain that is depression. No matter what: "You exist, therefore you matter." Don't give up on yourself.

CHAPTER 4

4 STEPS TO HEAL HEAD AND NECK PAIN

STEP 1:
PRACTICE LOVING-KINDNESS

I can tell you from experience that after turning inward to witness the mind and the body, I struggled a lot. Instead of allowing thoughts to pass and observing without judgment, I discovered attachment to high levels of mental and physical pain. No matter how hard I tried, I seemed to lack control over my inner world. I beat myself up for not being able to think more positively. This led to feeling trapped inside hurtful thoughts and a pained body for a long time.

It took decades of practice to observe my inner world with kindness. One day I noticed that I was extending a prayer for all beings everywhere to be happy and free, but excluding myself. I thought I didn't deserve happiness or freedom. This inner battle of unworthiness held me back from healing.

You don't have to wait decades. Start to treat your inner world with kindness right now. Make two columns: one for negative thoughts and one for positive ones. Write the negative stories that your mind repeats on one side and the opposite kind of words on the other. Here are a few of the stories my mind enjoys devising to make me feel bad about my pain:

Negative Thoughts	**Positive Thoughts**
I'm worthless.	*It's okay to ask for help.*
I can't do anything right.	*I'm doing the best I can right now.*
I'm always hurting myself.	*I can move with grace and strength.*
I need to stop wasting money on myself.	*Every time I pay for self-care, I am supporting a person in the healing profession.*
I am a selfish, privileged, piece of trash.	*I can take one step today to care for myself.*
I hate how sensitive I am.	*My sensitivities remind me to treat myself and others with love and respect.*
The healing arts make me weak.	*Yoga Therapy and Foundation Training give me the mobility I need to feel good daily, which allows me to serve others with more grace.*

CHAPTER 4: 4 STEPS TO HEAL HEAD AND NECK PAIN

Negative Thoughts	Positive Thoughts
I'm a waste of space.	I give back by helping others feel good.
I don't deserve a massage.	Massage helps me relax and release stress.
All this self-love crap is a waste of time; I'll always be broken.	The time I have committed to self-care has led to me being drug-free, to feeling better, to being strong, active, and to trusting that I am enough.

Negative Thoughts	Positive Thoughts

Whenever I find my mind running wild with negative thoughts, I know I am in an old holding pattern, and I need to practice loving-kindness to move out of it. This is when I return to the second column and practice kindness toward myself and others.

If you struggle with this concept of self-love and positive thoughts, it might be helpful to know that it's not your fault. It's your programming or your head injury. It's what you learned growing up or it's how your brain is reacting to a brain injury. Your brain is doing the best it can to help you, but sometimes the wires get crossed in an unhelpful way. Changing the negative loops in the brain isn't easy, but it is possible thanks to the neuroplasticity of the brain.

By choosing a positive thought from your pain-free list to replace the negative thoughts, you are rewiring your brain one thought at a time. This is an ancient practice that can be found in the Yoga Sutras of Patanjali in sutra 2.33: "When you are disturbed by unwholesome negative thoughts or emotions, cultivation of their opposites promotes self-control and firmness in the precepts." If you struggle with this and need help, a cognitive behavioral therapist can help rewire your brain. You don't have to do this work alone.

Place your positive thoughts somewhere you will see them. Create a calendar reminder in your phone that reminds you daily to to focus on developing more loving-kindness. Know that whatever comes up, you are not alone. You are not a mess. Your existence matters. You matter. Your life experiences matter. Your pain matters. Your pain can be transformed. You are not broken; even if your heart has been broken, you are still whole. You don't have to fight with yourself or anyone else. You have some challenges to overcome, and you can do that more easily if you observe the mind with kindness, and have it focus on healing. You deserve to feel better by focusing on loving-kindness for all beings, including yourself. You can access a five minute daily meditation to help you set the intention of loving-kindness toward self and others @ getwellwithdanielle.com/blog/lovingkindnessmeditation or @ https://youtu.be/jg-LwoJP1R4.

STEP 2:
IDENTIFY THE PAIN AND JOURNAL IT

Below you'll see two charts, the first is an example, and the second is for you to fill out. In the first column, write how the pain in your head and neck feels. In the second, write what you do that increases the pain. In the third, write what you do, or can do, to decrease the pain. If you don't know, leave it blank, and fill it in after you've gone through all four steps. Think about your pain as a mystery that needs to be solved— you get to investigate, gather the clues, and discover new ways to heal.

Here's my example chart:

What does the head and neck pain feel like?	What increases the pain?	What decreases the pain?
Constant tension and sharp pain at the base of my head.	Holding excessive downward facing dogs in yoga.	Practicing Founders from Foundation Training.
Headache radiates behind my eyes.	Sleeping on my belly.	Holding forward folds for a short time.
Neck and shoulders ache.	Looking down when I walk.	Resting in childs pose.
Sharp pain goes into the back of my eyes.	Not moving and being lazy.	Practicing gentle back extension exercises.

EMPOWERED CHOICES: A GUIDE TO HEALING HEAD & NECK PAIN

What does the head and neck pain feel like?	What increases the pain?	What decreases the pain?
Can't look over my shoulder without pain.	Receiving deep tissue massage.	Performing the joint freeing series regularly.
Constant pressure in my head and neck.	Hating myself for having injuries.	Practicing loving-kindness meditations and holding my phone up when I text.
Achey, dull, sharp, it keeps changing.	Being down on myself for not being able to hold plank, downward-facing dog, and for basically sucking at yoga.	Giving myself grace, practicing poses that feel strengthening, doing what I can, and Not comparing myself to others.
Sharp nerve pain in my neck when I move my head.	Stretching and everything I try on my own.	Receiving CranioSacral Therapy or getting a Chiropractic adjustment.

If you're having trouble filling out these three columns, sit in silence with your body and feel where the pain is and where it isn't. Imagine you're checking your cabinets to see what food you have and what food you don't. No judgment; it is what it is. Let's say you have an abundance of chips and nuts and brownie mixes, but no pasta and no rice. Take notice of the empty places in the cabinet, not just what you have, but also where there is room for more.

CHAPTER 4: 4 STEPS TO HEAL HEAD AND NECK PAIN

Scan your body the same way. Identify where there is consistent pain, the kind that comes and goes but is always returning with a constant annoyance and limitation. Are there any thoughts connected to the pain? Write it all down. You'll be able to solve the mysterious nature of your pain by writing down what you identify. Does the painful area feel stiff, achey, bound, sharp, dull, or unstable? Once you've taken inventory of your pain, figure out what is increasing your pain. Answer some of these questions below.

- Do you sit too much with bad posture? ❏ Yes ❏ No

- Are you at a computer too much with no stretch breaks? ❏ Yes ❏ No

- Are you a new parent holding a new baby all day? ❏ Yes ❏ No

- Do you have a labor-intensive job? ❏ Yes ❏ No

- How do you sleep?
  ❏ Stomach   ❏ Side   ❏ Back

- Does your head and neck pain feel worse in the morning? ❏ Yes ❏ No

- Does stress bring the pain on? ❏ Yes ❏ No

- If so, when do you notice it's worse?

_____

_____

_____

- Are there any other repetitive motions you are doing that could be aggravating your head and neck pain? ❏ Yes ❏ No

- If so, what do you think it is that's bothering your head and neck pain?

  _____
  _____
  _____

- Do you have pain from an old concussion or whiplash injury that you've never treated?   ❑ Yes   ❑ No

- If you have an exercise routine, how do you feel when you're working out?

  _____
  _____
  _____

- How do you feel after you work out?

  _____
  _____

- What kind of work and movement do you spend the majority of your time doing?

  _____
  _____
  _____

Now that you've filled out these questions go ahead and fill in the chart below. Any of the questions that you circled yes to need to be added to the second column below. If sleeping or working out is increasing your pain, add that to the chart as well.

What does the head and neck pain feel like?

_____
_____
_____
_____
_____

What increases the pain?

_____
_____
_____
_____
_____

What decreases the pain?

_____
_____
_____
_____
_____

Here's a quick example of someone who is increasing their current neck pain and what they can do to decrease it:

Let's call this person Sean. He works primarily on a computer and is constantly on his cell phone. He spends most of his time looking down toward the computer or down at the phone. After 10+ years at the same job, the muscles in his neck have learned to look down when he walks, when he works out, and when he does any other activity outside of work. On top of that, his range of motion is limited, and his neck feels stiff everyday. Some days he is in excruciating pain, other days it's manageable, but it isn't getting better.

The most obvious choice Sean can make is to raise his computer to eye level, so it better supports his posture since this is how he spends the majority of his time. He can also take stretch breaks throughout the day to increase the range of motion in his neck, to keep it from getting worse. Sean and other people living with head and neck pain will benefit from the simple practice of lengthening through all sides of the neck and focusing the gaze straight ahead. You can do this while working, driving, walking, really anytime. This will help train the neck to return to its natural curve when you're not staring at a computer or a cell phone.

To the best of your ability, avoid movements that make it worse. I know this sounds obvious, but so many people feel pain from a specific motion and keep doing the same movement anyway, saying, "It hurts when I do this." Stop doing what hurts.

Now, how do you decrease the pain?

First, feel the space beyond the pain. In other words, become aware of the wholeness of your entire being, rather than just the parts that feel terrible. Choose one thing you can do to change a habit that is making your pain worse or keeping it the same. Add this new habit to the new positive thought you are working with. It is one thing to have injuries that limit your physical body; it's another to have a mind that identifies wholeheartedly with those physical limitations. If you have a current exercise routine, does it alleviate the tension in your head and neck? If so, which movements lessen the pain? If you don't have a routine yet, that's okay. You'll get there soon.

If Sean were my client, I would advise him to invest in a simple S-curve back massager. The one I use is the Body Back Buddy Elite. This tool allows you to hold a trigger point, breathe into it, and help your muscle tension decrease. I would also direct him to the Top 3 Best Exercises for Relieving Head & Neck Pain at my blog https://www.getwellwithdanielle.com/blog/neck-exercises

Your last two columns may not be full of ideas yet, but as you read through this book, you'll have lightbulb moments. Keep track of the activities, people, and thoughts that increase the good pain and decrease the bad pain—learning to listen is half of the battle.

We all face hardship, injuries, and pain. Some of us more than others. Whether physical, emotional, or traumatic, your pain is a part of your human experience. Your relationship to your pain is a choice. For me, I found that the more I ignored the physical pain and focused on the emotional pain, the worse the physical pain became. When I addressed the physical pain, the emotional pain lessened.

STEP 3:
PRACTICE EXERCISES TO INCREASE A HEALTHY RANGE OF MOTION

The feel-good and strengthening exercises in this book are meant to minimize and lessen pain from chronic head and neck injuries. They will build muscular flexibility, strength, balance, and stability. If one of them doesn't feel right, try another until you find the one that works for your body. This experimentation will add to the puzzle pieces you're gathering and give you a clearer picture of how to heal.

If none of them work then right away, you'll know something deeper is going on and that you need to seek professional help before proceeding. If that's you, flip to chapter 11 or 12 to and explore the movement options and practitioner that sounds like the best fit.. Looking for feel-good exercises? A practitioner who is trained in Therapeutic or restorative yoga is the best place to start.

These exercises will build up your weak muscles. It's important to approach them slowly. Try a couple of reps daily and, if it feels good, try a few more. If it feels challenging, that's okay too. If it feels challenging and it's aggravating the current pain in the area, flip to chapter 12 and find a trainer who has practice in the strength training that sounds most appealing to you. You can also identify physical therapy or chiropractic care, which may be covered by your insurance.

The exercises are split into five sections: neck, shoulder, core, back extension, and full body exercises that pull everything together for optimal head and neck health. Photos and directions show the movement and explain how to practice it. Want more direct instructions? Check out https://www.getwellwithdanielle.com/head-neck-pain

STEP 4:
FIND A HEALING PROFESSIONAL

It's important to be aware of the various types of personal training, yoga, and massage. Although I will focus on these three healing options, many other professionals and forms of movement can help you heal. My hope is that you will feel empowered to follow your intuition, reach out to professionals, and step into living a healthier happier life. The best place to start is to contact professionals who have been recommended. Next, read testimonials. Notice who you feel drawn to and connect with them.

Most healing professionals have been trained in various modalities and combine them. If you feel drawn to a specific technique, tell your therapist, and they can focus on what will best serve you. Some services, such as CranioSacral therapy and Foundation Training, require specialized training, so be sure to find someone who practices the modalities you're looking for. For example: don't seek out someone who gives deep tissue massage or Rolfing massage if you're looking for a light-touch massage. If you don't want to be naked, draped with sheets, and have your skin massaged with oil or lotion, seek out a sports or Thai massage therapist; this way you can stay fully clothed.

If you're looking for a professional who is covered under insurance, find out if your insurance covers physical therapy, chiropractic care, and/or acupuncture. Find the practitioners who check off the most boxes for the services you seek. I go into this in more detail in Chapter 8: Finding a Healing Professional.

If your mind has convinced you that your pain doesn't matter, that you don't deserve to heal, that everyone else's needs come first, that you don't have time for yourself, then your mind is doing a disservice to you and to the people who are waiting to help you get well. Revisit step one and create a positive thought that will propel you to find the right support.

CHAPTER 5

FEEL-GOOD RELIEF TIPS

These tips speak for themselves; they feel good. If they don't feel good, don't practice them. If you're on a lot of medication, if you've suffered from a recent injury and need medical advice, or if you're unsure about any of these tips, ask your trusted doctor of physical therapy, doctor of chiropractic care, doctor of acupressure, or your primary care doctor if they think it will be beneficial for you.

Most importantly, listen to your body's intelligence—it will tell you what feels right. I keep repeating this concept because it is not easy to be still and to observe. It is possible though, and I promise that the more you practice, the easier it will become to drop into your body's natural ability to feel better.

Some of the suggested creams, pills, and injections in this chapter I have used with success; others I have heard of from clients, family, and friends. My intention is to share a broad list, so you can find what will help you. These feel-good tips are simple ways to practice loving kindness toward your injury.

Tip #1: Ice or heat the injured area.

Ice and heat are not interchangeable. Ice will lessen inflammation and swelling by pulling blood away from the injured area. Heat will relax the muscles and bring blood flow back to the muscles. General suggestions for ice or heat are 10-15 minutes on the injured area every 1-4 hours. Don't exceed 20 minutes of ice or heat. Personally, I have an aversion to ice. I hate being cold, but every time I've pulled a muscle from pushing my body to go beyond what it's capable of (which happens less these days, but still happens), ice helps lessen the pain from inflammation. I always turn to heat though because warmth sounds good and feels good at first. For my body, I almost always need to follow up with ice. The heat brings too much blood flow to the already irritated area and doesn't ultimately help it feel better. Write down how you feel after you've used the ice or heat. Did the pain lessen? If so, for how long? If not, try something else.

Tip # 2: Find a cream that works for you.

When you have achy joints, a pinched nerve, a muscle spasm, chronic neck pain, or a headache that's coming from neck tension, it can be helpful to apply a therapeutic cream. It is soothing to the muscles and the nervous system to receive recurring touch that is relaxing. Each cream relaxes the muscles in a different way.

If something doesn't work for you, give it to someone you think may benefit from using it, and try something else. A quick Google search will elicit a long list of creams that may help, but it is important to consider the different ingredients and which ones will help you the most. Your skin is the largest organ in your body, and it is going to absorb whatever you put on it. For this reason, you may need to explore your options. Here are a few ways to narrow your choices:

1. Read the ingredients. If the ingredients aren't easily accessible, move on to a product that is more transparent.

CHAPTER 5: FEEL-GOOD RELIEF TIPS

2. Notice if there are additives or parabens. Not all additives are bad, but if you're not sure and don't have the time to research it, it's easier to find a product with ingredients that you know will help. There are mixed reviews on parabens, but these 5 types of parabens have been banned in Europe because they are believed to be endocrine disruptors: isopropylparaben, isobutylparaben, phenylparaben, benzylparaben, & pentylparaben. When in doubt, I look to see what Europe is doing because, if they are banning certain ingredients, it's likely for a legitimate reason. If the first ingredient is water, it isn't bad, it just means that water is the majority of what will be in it. Personally, I'd rather choose a product that has one of the ingredients below as the first ingredient listed. When trying something new, use a small amount to be sure you aren't allergic.

3. If you're sensitive to smells, stick to the first two options below. If you are unsure about scents, go to Pharmaca, Whole Foods, or another speciality store to sniff out products. The list below is where I start when I have achy joints, a pinched nerve, a muscle spasm, chronic neck pain, or a headache from neck tension:

   - Arnica Montana cream, gel, or oil is a flower extract. I use the Boion Brand for the cream and the gel. It has 7% Arnica. I use the PipingRock brand of Arnica Montana oil, and I like to mix it with other essential oils.

   - Traumeel is a wonderful cream that has Arnica and additional plant medicine included in it. It has a light scent, and I love it. My 80 year-old aunt also likes it.

   - My choice of essential oils for relieving head and neck pain are DoTerra Lavender, DeepBlue, or Serenity blend. The DeepBlue is my go-to for neck pain. You won't find these products in stores. If you haven't tried it, I recommend trying the DeepBlueRub samples to make sure the smell isn't too strong. The rub is cheaper than the oil, but it's also watered down and has additional ingredients.

- Tiger Balm Ultra- 11 % menthol and 11% camphor is very relaxing to the muscles, giving a warm cooling effect with a strong scent. There are many products that can be found on the Tiger Balm website, but be sure to check all the inactive ingredients. I don't recommend products with added dyes and parabens. This is why the Ultra is my go-to.

I haven't tried the options below yet, but I know people who have found relief from them. New CBD and THC creams are available, and people can benefit from different combinations of them. It can be helpful to find a dispensary that works with a medical lab to find the best option for you. In general, I search for the option with the most CBD; just know that this is more expensive.

- Pain Pain Go Away from Good Jane: I've heard that this CBD rub works wonders. Plus, the product tube is 100% recyclable. It has 500 mg of broad spectrum hemp or CBD, Arnica, ginger, and other helpful plant medicine.
- Blosum: This contains 500 mg of CBD with Arnica and other helpful ingredients.
- The VooDoo Lab's active ingredient is Trolamine Salicylate 10%. There are some plant extracts in this product, such as Arnica and chamomile. It also has MSM in it, which is helpful for achy joints. (More on this under Feel Good Tip #5).
- Anti-inflammatory cream from a doctor.

Tip #3: Try an epsom salt bath or a sensory deprivation float tank.

- Take a bath. Add a cup or two of Epsom salt or essential oils for relaxation and relief.
- Try a float tank, where you float freely for an hour or 90 minutes. You can find these with a simple Google search. This can accelerate the recovery from an injury, boost the immune system by allowing you to fully relax, and more.

Tip #4: Try a few simple self-massage techniques for the head and neck. (More detailed descriptions and a pin and stretch video can be found on my website http://getwellwithdanielle.com/blog)

- Place your fingers on the bottom of your neck and make small circles in each direction. Slowly move the circles up along the sides of the neck. Press your fingers in toward each other as they circle up the sides of the neck until you reach the base of the skull. Take your thumbs to the base of your skull and wrap your hands around your head. Then pull upward with the thumbs. This creates traction and allows space between the head and the top neck vertebrae.
- Place the heels of your hands on the sides of your head near the upper portion of the head. Gently press the hands in toward each other with a light pressure. and lift the heels of your hands up toward the ceiling. This subtle technique helps alleviate head and neck pain.

Tip #5: Try acupuncture, chiropractic care, or physical therapy.

Many health insurance plans now cover acupuncture, chiropractic care, or physical therapy. Check with your insurance company to see what they cover. At many community clinics, acupuncturists offer discounted rates; some chiropractors offer a free first time consultation. Not sure what to look for or where to start? Skip ahead to chapter 8.

Tip #6: Sample alternative medicines for head and neck pain.
If the pain in your neck is coming from inflammation, the following alternatives may help reduce it. If you're on other medications or aren't sure about how much to take, ask a trusted doctor.

- Ginger capsules
- Arnica pills
- Traumeel pills
- IBUPROFEN or Aspirin
- MSM (a chemical found in humans, animals, and plants): I've known people who find immediate relief from taking a small amount each day. Anytime I have achy joints, this is my go-to supplement, and it reduces the pain almost immediately. I stop taking it when I don't feel the pain.

Tip #7: Try injections.
 In more severe cases, you may need to find an injection to help relieve your head or neck pain.

- Platelet Rich Plasma therapy takes a small amount of a patient's blood and injects it into the injured site to strengthen the body's natural healing abilities.
- Cortisone shots are a corticosteroid injection that can reduce pain and inflammation. I know people who need only one for the entire year to increase their quality of life.
- Ajoyvi is a migraine medication that you can inject monthly or once every 3 months. One of my clients went from having at

least 10-12 migraines per month to 5 migraines in 3 months. Ajovy is very expensive and most practitioners/insurance companies require you to have 10-15 migraines a month and that you try several pharmaceutical treatments before they give it to you.

Tip #8: Practice a daily mantra that encourages loving kindness toward yourself and others. One of the most powerful mantras I have used is Om Shanti Shanti Shanti. Om symbolizes creation, preservation, and destruction. It represents God, the Universe, a Higher Power, the invisible force that connects all of us. Shanti stands for Peace.

- Sit in a cross legged position or on the edge of a chair with your spine elongated or lay flat on your back with your feet on the floor and the knees bent.
- Set a timer for 1, 5, or 10 minutes.
- Place your right pinky finger together with your right thumb.
- Silently say, "Om, Shanti, Shanti, Shanti."
- Take your ring finger and thumb together and repeat again, Om, Shanti, Shanti, Shanti.
- Change your fingers and switch to your left hand, beginning each time with the pinky and thumb together.
- If that feels too complicated, get meditation beads, and each time you repeat the mantra, move to a new bead.
- This practice will help keep your mind focused on each repetition. Each time the mind wanders, come back to the mantra and the beads.
- As you get more comfortable, hold the intention of peace, calm, and serenity for yourself and others with each repetition.

CHAPTER 6

IDENTIFY GOOD VS. BAD PAIN

Billions of dollars are invested in creating drugs to reduce pain. Instead of paying more money to pharmaceutical companies, why not explore where your pain is coming from, decipher what is good pain, what is bad pain, what is accumulated pain from previous injuries, what pain can be worked through with manual manipulation and movement therapy, and what is simply discomfort from living in a human body?

Good Pain	**Bad Pain**
<ul><li>Moves out of the body.</li><li>Dissipates after an exercise practice or a few days.</li><li>Tends to feel like growing pains.</li><li>Uncomfortable, but not limiting.</li><li>Muscular Burn.</li></ul>	<ul><li>Sharp</li><li>Numb</li><li>Reoccurring</li><li>Tingly</li><li>Achy</li><li>Hurts in joints</li><li>Limits your range of motion</li><li>Leads to bruising</li><li>A warning sign that something is wrong</li></ul>

An example of good pain: A burning sensation in your muscles when receiving a deep tissue massage. As long as you can breathe comfortably into the sensations and continue to communicate with the therapist, it's likely good. This kind of pain comes from places in the connective tissue that are bound and need to be broken apart in order to function better. If it's good pain, it may be a little sore for a day or two, but overall you'll feel better. (If you're tensing other muscles, want to run from the therapist, or find deep bruising after, it's bad pain.)

An example of bad pain: When you drop your ear toward your shoulder and get a sharp pain into the head or neck or down into the shoulder. This kind of pain usually comes from an injury or repetitive stress. It happens when a nerve is pinched or a bone is out of place. If you continue to aggravate this pain, it will likely cause more discomfort and not alleviate what's happening in your head and neck. Bad pain is generally a warning that something is wrong; it's sharp, quick, tingly, numb, and aches. It returns often. It's the kind of pain you experience right after a car accident, injury, or from repetitive stress. It's the kind of pain that needs time to heal and recover. Not the kind of pain you push through. The kind that tells you something is out of alignment or off balance. It often returns in the same place when you run, sit, drive, or do other daily activities.

Bad pain hurts and limits your range of motion. Good pain is uncomfortable, not limiting. When practicing yoga, good pain is when you feel the muscles soften and lengthen as you breathe. When practicing strength training, good pain burns because it is building new muscle. The key is to feel the stretch or contraction in the right muscles, not in your joints, tendons, and ligaments. For example, when you drop one ear to one shoulder and feel a stretch along the length of the muscleon the other side of the neck. Or possibly youfeel restricted; your head doesn't move very far and it feels stiff. That's okay— over time it will loosen, and your range of motion will increase— one breath at a time.

I used to push through bad pain, and it resulted in making me feel worthless, weak, and broken. Now when I feel pain, I determine if it is coming from weakness, inactivity, too much activity, stress, an old injury, an old painful storyline, or a combination. Then I apply the four steps to healing head and neck pain, and I feel better.

IS IT A GOOD OR BAD STORYLINE?

In my experience, the body can't be separated from the mind and the spirit. It's important to become aware of the storylines your mind is feeding you. Are the narratives creating more pain or lessening it? Here are the Painful Stories I hold in my head and neck:

Bad Storylines	Good Storylines
My voice doesn't matter.	My voice matters. I exist; therefore, I matter.
I'm an idiot.	I am intelligent. I have gifts, I have resources, I have healing tools, and I am ready to share them.
What I have to say doesn't really matter, just suck it up.	This guide to healing head and neck pain will be a resource for myself and others to heal faster.
I have to do everything on my own.	I ask for help, and I receive it with grace.
I'm going to fail at this too.	I am flawed. That's what makes me human, and I'm okay with that.

Bad Storylines	Good Storylines
I don't deserve to be treated kindly.	I treat myself with loving kindness. I stand with grace and I move with ease into the new chapters of my life.
Nobody cares that I'm hurting.	I care that I am hurting. I listen to my body, my mind, my heart. I honor it and follow its intelligence.
Complaining is the only way for me to be heard.	My voice is heard by sharing stories. I am a courageous storyteller.

These thoughts are followed by descriptive stories that keep me believing them. When they are in charge, I feel pain--trapped in my chest, shoulders, and neck. I twist and stretch and pull and push and wiggle and move to try to get rid of it, but it's energetic pain. It's the painful voices in my head and in my body that I can't escape because they are locked inside. I feel crooked. These twisted stories pull me in opposite directions.

Part of me thinks I need these wicked stories to feel alive, to feel connected to suffering, to feel anything. The other part of me thinks these stories are trash and need to be dumped off and washed away. I need new stories to uplift me, to unravel the pain, to move forward with grace and ease. That's where the New Stories come in handy. Here's a blank chart for you to fill out.

CHAPTER 6: IDENTIFY GOOD VS. BAD PAIN

Bad Storylines	Good Storylines

CHAPTER 7

EXERCISES FOR HEAD AND NECK HEALTH

By practicing the exercises offered in this chapter, you will increase the stability, mobility, and strength in your neck, and as a result, your head and neck pain will diminish. Begin with the first exercise in each section. They are organized from easiest to most difficult. Ideally, you'll find a routine that feels good and is easy to practice regularly. If it feels challenging, start with fewer reps and progress slowly.

At the end of each section, you will find a suggested pose for relaxation. This can be paired with any and all of the exercises in this book.

If pain persists and you find these simple movements worsen current pain, seek a movement professional. Find someone who specializes in strengthening neck muscles: a seasoned yoga instructor, a Foundation Training instructor, a skilled Pilates instructor, a physical therapist, or a chiropractor. For more detailed descriptions of these professionals, flip to Chapter 12.

Alternatively, you can find me online at getwellwithdanielle.com. I have a 6 Week Manage & Relieve Head & Neck Pain Program available to support you in creating a safe weekly movement practice. I'd love to support you.

The exercises below are simple and safe. They teach you to get in touch with the wisdom of your body. You'll get clear about the movements that hurt your head and neck, and the ones that make it stronger. If you've had a recent injury, give yourself time to recover before practicing these exercises.

NECK EXERCISES

The neck exercises below include an isometric contraction to strengthen and stabilize your deep neck muscles, and various ways to rotate the neck to increase neck mobility. These movements will help imprint a healthy range of motion in the neck so that looking over your shoulder when driving will get easier and the fear of throwing out your neck will diminish. In all of these poses, it is important to create space at the base of the skull where the nerves pass through the foramen magnum. Be mindful of how your head and neck feel during and after these exercises.

CHAPTER 7: EXERCISES FOR HEAD AND NECK HEALTH

#1: Practice Isometric Contraction
4-8 reps, 1 set/day

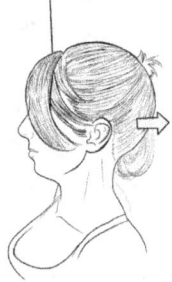 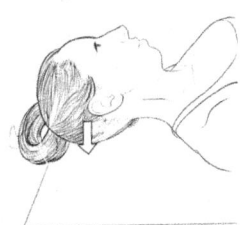

- Lie flat on the back or sit up against a wall.
- Open and close the jaw a few times.
- Relax the tongue from the roof of the mouth.
- Feel the length along all four sides of the neck.
- Breathe in and feel the length along all sides of the neck.
- Breathe out and press the back of the head straight into the floor or the wall.
- Create space around the hole at the base of the skull, the foramen magnum.
- Relax and repeat.

* This can also be done in the car, even when stuck in traffic by pressing your head against the headrest.

#keepingtrack

These questions will help you discover which postures are helping and which ones to stay away from, for now.

During this exercise, I felt _____

After this exercise, I felt _____

#2: Practice Neck Rotation
4-8 reps–1 set/day

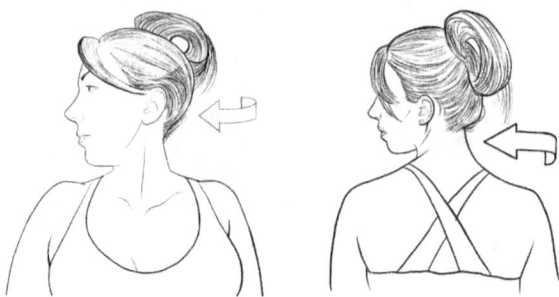

- Lay on your back with your feet on the floor. To make this more challenging, sit upright in a chair.
- Inhale lengthen all sides of the neck, exhale, and rotate your head to the right.
- Inhale and bring the head back to center. Imagine you can touch the crown of your head to the ceiling. This will help elongate the neck.
- Exhale, rotate the head to the left. This completes one rep.

*Remember: keep your chin parallel with the floor.

#keepingtrack

During this exercise, I felt _____

_____

_____

After this exercise, I felt _____

_____

_____

CHAPTER 7: EXERCISES FOR HEAD AND NECK HEALTH

#3: Practice Lateral Flexion
5 reps on each side—1 set/day

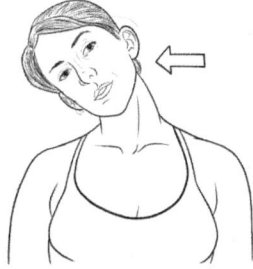 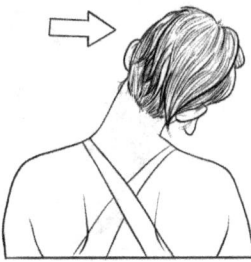

- Sit upright on a chair or sit upright on the floor.
- Inhale to lengthen all sides of the neck and exhale drop the right ear toward the right shoulder.
- Inhale bring the head back to center and exhale, drop the left ear to the left shoulder.
- Do your best to keep your gaze focused straight ahead so that the head doesn't rotate toward the floor.
- Move the head as though it is swaying side to side in water, without force.

*If you experience a sharp pain on either side of the neck when you practice this posture, flip to the self-massage Tip #4 in Chapter 5 Feel Good Relief Tips. Or follow the link for the pin and stretch technique mentioned at the beginning of Tip #4. If that doesn't relieve the pain, find a professional to massage your neck.

#keepingtrack

During this exercise, I felt _____

_____

After this exercise, I felt _____

_____

#4 Practice Lateral Flexion with Rotation
1-3 reps—1 set a day

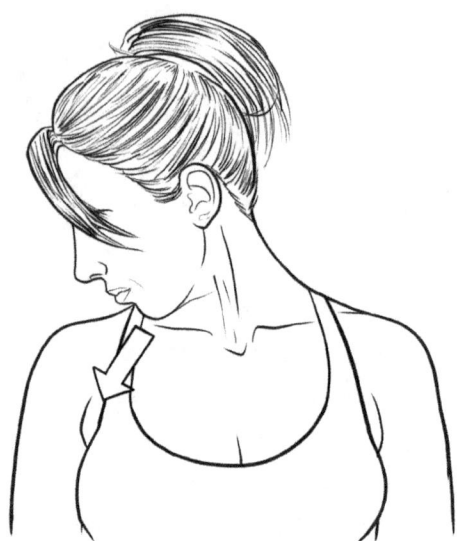

- Sit upright on a chair or sit upright on the floor.
- Inhale to lengthen all sides of the neck and exhale drop the right ear toward the right shoulder.
- Hold this position for 3-4 breaths allowing the head to drop a tiny bit further with each exhale.
- On your fourth exhale tilt the chin toward the armpit and gaze down at the right inner elbow.
- Take 3-4 breaths here.
- Drop the chin toward the chest, look down toward the belly button, and breathe into the upper back.
- Take 3-4 breaths here.
- On your inhale, lift the head back to an upright position.
- Inhale to lengthen all sides of the neck and exhale. Drop the left ear toward the left shoulder.

CHAPTER 7: EXERCISES FOR HEAD AND NECK HEALTH

- Hold this position for 3-4 breaths, allowing the head to drop a tiny bit further with each exhale.
- On your fourth exhale, tilt the chin toward the armpit and gaze down at the left inner elbow.
- Take 3-4 breaths here.
- Drop the chin toward the chest, look down toward the belly button, and breathe into the upper back.
- Take 3-4 here.
- On your inhale, lift the head back to an upright position.

*With each exhale remember to relax the jaw, the face, and any tension you may be holding in the shoulders.

#keepingtrack

During this exercise, I felt _____
_____
_____
_____
_____
_____
_____

After this exercise, I felt _____
_____
_____
_____
_____
_____
_____

#5 Practice Neck Extension & Flexion
1-3 reps—1 set a day

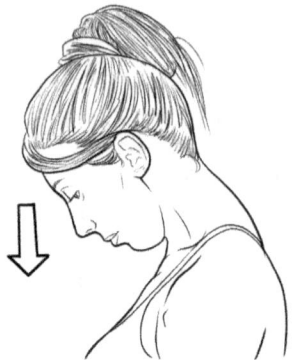
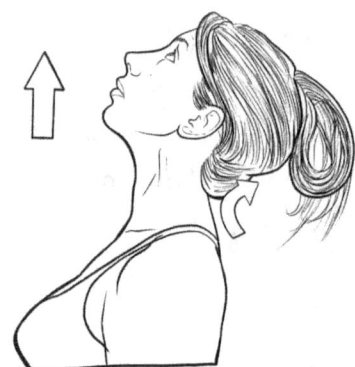

- Sit upright on a chair or stand with your feet hip distance apart.
- Inhale to lengthen all sides of the neck and begin to look up toward the ceiling, increasing the arch in the back of the neck.
- Exhale, lowering the chin toward the chest.
- Repeat.

*Be careful not to collapse at the base of the skull. The purpose of this exercise is to lengthen and strengthen the muscles along the back of the neck, especially the small muscles at the base of the skull that help hold your head up.

#keepingtrack

During this exercise, I felt _____

_____

After this exercise, I felt _____

_____

#6 Relax and Support Neck Extension
1-3 minutes - 1 set/day.

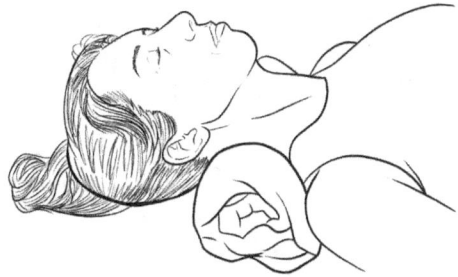

- Fold a body towel lengthwise in half to double its thickness.
- Roll it up the way you would a yoga mat.
- Lay flat on your back, and place the towel under the neck to support the natural extension of the neck. Make sure the back of your head touches the floor.
- You can start with a small roll if that feels best and increase the size of the roll over time as your neck extension increases.

*Remember: any exercises that increase your current pain need to be avoided. Give yourself time to rebuild muscular stability and to learn about the different sensations you're feeling. Track how you feel during and after the exercises.

#keepingtrack

During this exercise, I felt _____

_____

After this exercise, I felt _____

_____

Create a workout just for you by saying how many reps felt good to practice and keep track below. If you don't think the exercise is helpful, put a line through the rep section for now.

Neck Exercises	Reps
Isometric Contraction	
Neck Rotation	
Lateral Flexion	
Lateral Flexion w/ Rotation	
Neck Extension and Neck Flexion	
Relax and Support Neck Extension	

SHOULDER EXERCISES

Why have I included exercises for the shoulders in a book about head and neck pain? Because a few muscles that connect to the skull and neck vertebrae also connect to the shoulder blade. When you release tension in the shoulders and create stability in the shoulder muscles, it helps the head move with more ease. The shoulder exercises below will strengthen postural muscles, which will help coax the neck into alignment.

Begin by practicing one of the three exercises below for one week. Keep track of what you feel during and after. If the exercise is helpful, stick with it, and add in one of the other two exercises. If it doesn't feel good, trade it out for a different one. Explore these various ways to move your shoulders, and enjoy the benefits of increased range of motion.

Practice Shoulder Retraction and Protraction
4-8 reps, 1 set/day.

3 Ways to Practice this Exercise:
#1. Rest on Back

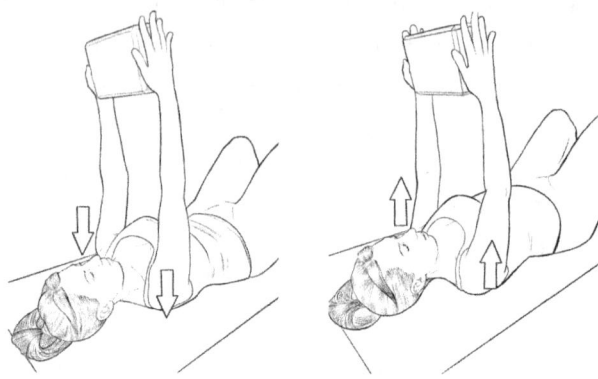

- Lie flat on your back.
- Extend arms up toward the ceiling so that the fingertips face the ceiling and the palms face each other.
- Exhale and press the shoulders down into the floor.
- Inhale and reach the fingertips up toward the ceiling.
- This will lift the shoulders away from the floor and begin to stretch and strengthen the muscles around the shoulder; this will in turn better support the neck.

#keepingtrack

During this exercise, I felt _____

_____

After this exercise, I felt _____

_____

CHAPTER 7: EXERCISES FOR HEAD AND NECK HEALTH

#2. All Fours

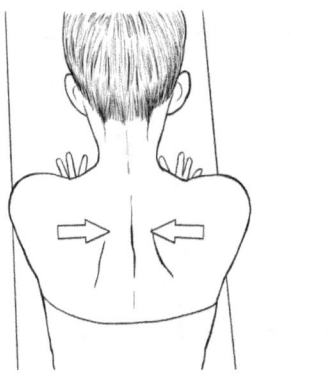 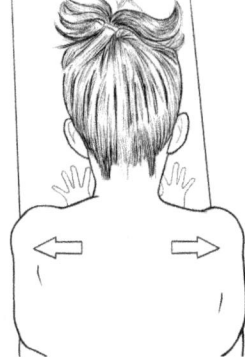

- Come onto all fours and align your hands under your shoulders and your knees under your hips.
- Inhale and drop the chest toward the floor, squeezing shoulder blades together.
- Exhale and spread the shoulder blades apart by pushing the hands into the ground and allowing the shoulder blades to press away from each other.

#keepingtrack

During this exercise, I felt _____
_____
_____
_____
_____

After this exercise, I felt _____
_____
_____
_____
_____

#3. Hands on Shoulders

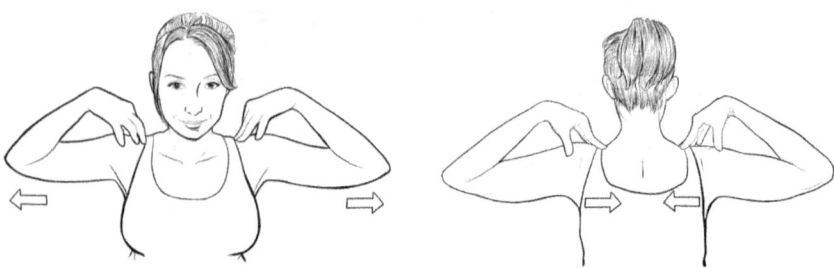

- Place your hands on your shoulders and lift the elbows out to the sides until they are at the height of the shoulders.
- Inhale and hug the shoulder blades together.
- Exhale. Bring the elbows forward and toward each other. Over time the elbows may touch as in the photo below.
- Be sure to lengthen across the chest and upper back before retracting the shoulder blades. As in the image below.

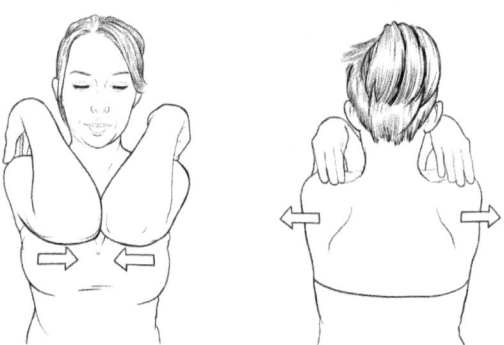

#keepingtrack

During this exercise, I felt _____
_____

After this exercise, I felt _____
_____

CHAPTER 7: EXERCISES FOR HEAD AND NECK HEALTH

Shoulder Circles
4-8 reps in each direction, 1 set/day
3 Ways to Practice this Exercise:
#1. Hands on Shoulders

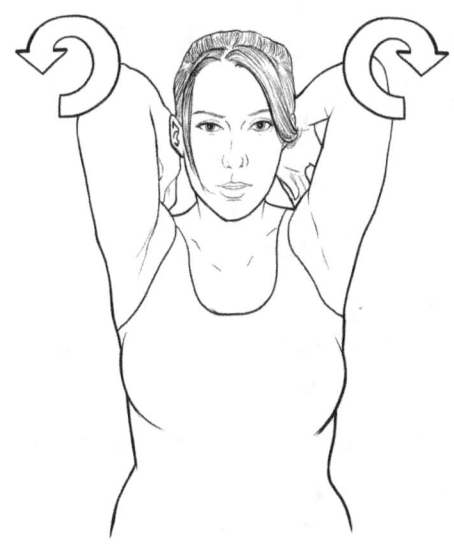

- Bring fingertips onto shoulders.
- As you inhale, bring the elbows forward and up toward the ceiling.
- On your exhale, bring the elbows wide and take them down toward the floor to complete the circle.
- This will take the shoulder blades into slight retraction.
- After you do a few in this direction, reverse it.

EMPOWERED CHOICES: A GUIDE TO HEALING HEAD & NECK PAIN

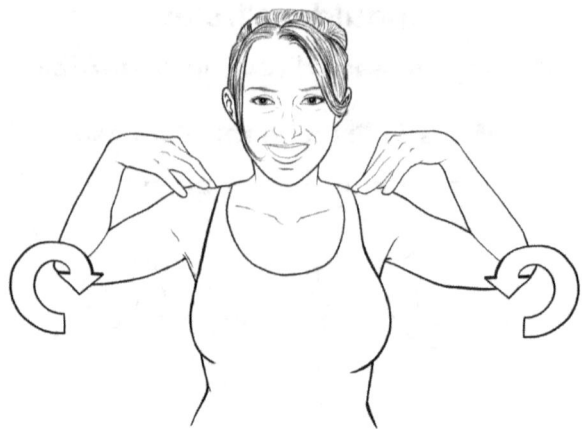

- Bring your fingertips onto your shoulders.
- As you inhale, bring your elbows down and up toward the ceiling. This will take the shoulder blades into slight retraction as you lift the elbows back and up.
- On your exhale, bring the elbows forward and down. The elbows may or may not touch, don't force it.
- Slowly increase your range of motion by practicing these daily.

#keepingtrack

During this exercise, I felt _____
_____
_____
_____
_____

After this exercise, I felt _____
_____
_____
_____
_____

CHAPTER 7: EXERCISES FOR HEAD AND NECK HEALTH

#2. Arms Out to Sides

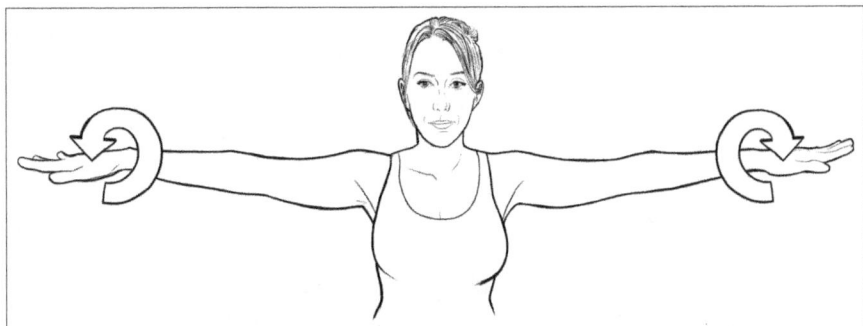

- Extend arms out to the sides.
- Make small circles forward and small circles backward with your arms.
- Imagine you are drawing circles on the side walls—these circles can eventually get bigger, and as they do you'll want to slow down your breathing.
- Inhale as the arms come up. Exhale as they come down.

#*keepingtrack*

During this exercise, I felt _____

_____

_____

_____

After this exercise, I felt _____

_____

_____

_____

#3. Foam Roll Shoulder Circles

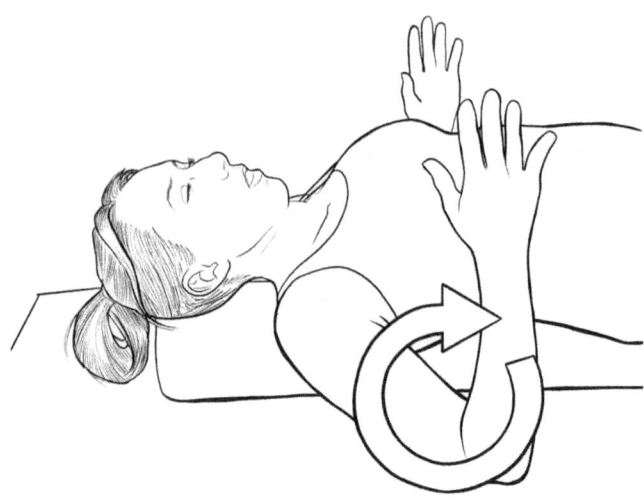

- Lay your entire back and head along a foam roller with your head on one side and your butt on the other.
- Bend your elbows and circle the shoulders forward for a few reps and backward for a few reps.

*You need a full length foam roller for this one.

#keepingtrack

During this exercise, I felt _____
_____
_____
_____

After this exercise, I felt _____
_____
_____
_____

CHAPTER 7: EXERCISES FOR HEAD AND NECK HEALTH

#3 RELAX with the Foam Roll Pec. Stretch
1-3 minutes, 1 set/day.

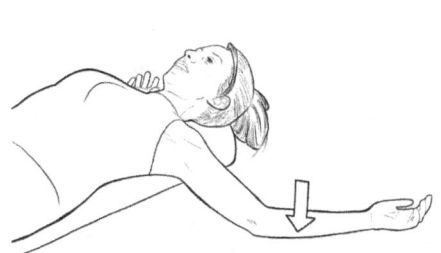
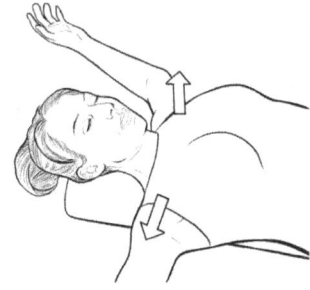

- This pose supports the relaxation of the shoulder blades and the opening of the chest.
- Sit on one side of the foam roller and rest your head on the other side, so that your entire back is resting on the foam roller.
- Bring arms out to the sides, so they are level with the shoulders. If this already feels like a big stretch across the chest, stick with this until you feel you can go further.
- To add on, bend the elbows so that you're making a goal post shape.
- Press the back of your ribs into the roller. Let your arms drop toward the floor, so the back of your forearms and the back of your hands eventually rest on the floor.

#keepingtrack

During this exercise, I felt _____

_____

After this exercise, I felt _____

_____

*Remember: Sharp pain feels different than fatigued or weak muscular pain, and it is usually a sign to back off. Constant dull pain can also be a sign to back off. If the pain isn't lessening after two weeks of consistent daily practice, ask yourself: are the exercises creating bad pain or good pain? Set aside the ones that add bad pain, and try a couple new ones. Think of this as adding more puzzle pieces to your healing journey; the picture may not be clear yet, but with each piece, you'll be one step closer to completing the puzzle.

Create a workout just for you by saying how many reps felt good to practice and keep track below. If you don't think the exercise is helpful, put a line through the rep section for now.

Shoulder Exercises	Reps
Retraction and Protraction 1. Rest on Back 2. All Fours 3. Hands on Shoulders	
Shoulder Circles 1. Hands on Shoulders 2. Arms Out to Sides 3. Foam Roll Shoulder Circles	
Relax with Foam Roll Pec. Stretch	

CHAPTER 7: EXERCISES FOR HEAD AND NECK HEALTH

CORE EXERCISES

For years, I focused on creating mobility in my neck, and because I had chronic neck pain, I couldn't even do something as basic as a crunch without pain. I didn't have a clue about how to wake up my core strength, and I didn't know it was connected to my neck pain. My entire journey of healing head and neck pain is realizing that all of the muscles and the pain experienced in the body is connected. There are literal connective tissues that wrap around muscles and organs and spread through the entire muscular system. This is basic knowledge to some people, but it took years before I discovered the myofascial connective tissues. All I knew was that I was too young to feel weak and in chronic pain. Where you are weak, you need to build strength. Where you are stiff, you need mobility and flexibility.

When core muscles are weak, the exercises here will help strengthen them. Don't worry: no sit ups and no straining the neck. They will awaken deep stomach muscles, relax neck muscles, and get your lower body to better support your upper body.

In all of the exercises, focus on keeping your head and neck relaxed, so your core muscles are the primary muscles being used. If any of these exercises strain your neck muscles, come back to them when you've built more strength, stability, and mobility from the other exercises.

These core exercises will also prepare your body to practice safe twists and back extensions, the next two sets of exercises.

Seated Pulsing Abs
3 reps–1 set/day
with 30 sec. rest between sets

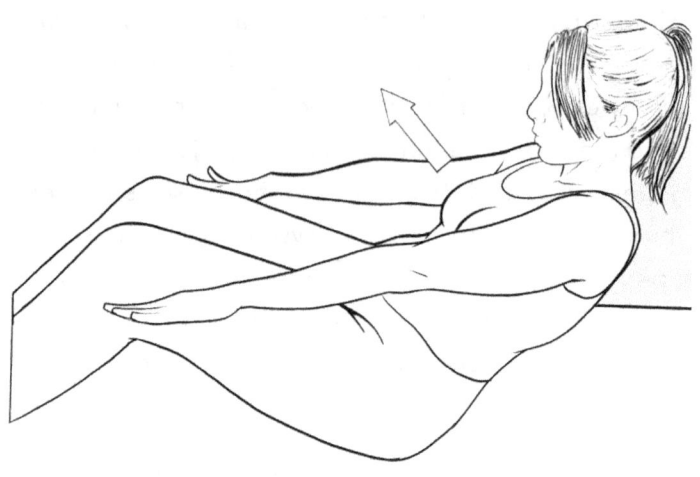

- Sit on the floor with knees bent in front. Hold onto the knees to lift the chest.
- Interlace the fingers, and bring the hands behind the head for support.
- Push the lowest part of the back toward the ball.
- Relax the head.
- Continue to roll until you feel the core quiver and shake.
- If your neck muscles feel stable enough, extend one arm forward and take a full breath.
- Inhale. Lift the arm up toward the ceiling and lift the gaze. Take a full breath here.
- Lower the arm back down.

CHAPTER 7: EXERCISES FOR HEAD AND NECK HEALTH

- Switch arms so that one hand is behind the head and the other arm is extended forward. Take a full breath here.
- Lift one arm up toward the ceiling, lift the gaze, and relax the head into the hand. Take a full breath here.
- Come up, hold onto the knees, lift the chest, and rest.
- Repeat.

*The most gentle way to wake up your abs is to use a pilates ball behind your low back. If you don't have one, try the exercise below.

#*keepingtrack*

During this exercise, I felt _____
_____
_____
_____
_____
_____
_____
_____
_____

After this exercise, I felt _____
_____
_____
_____
_____
_____
_____
_____
_____

Slow Roll Down
3 reps–1 set/day
with a 30 sec. rest between sets

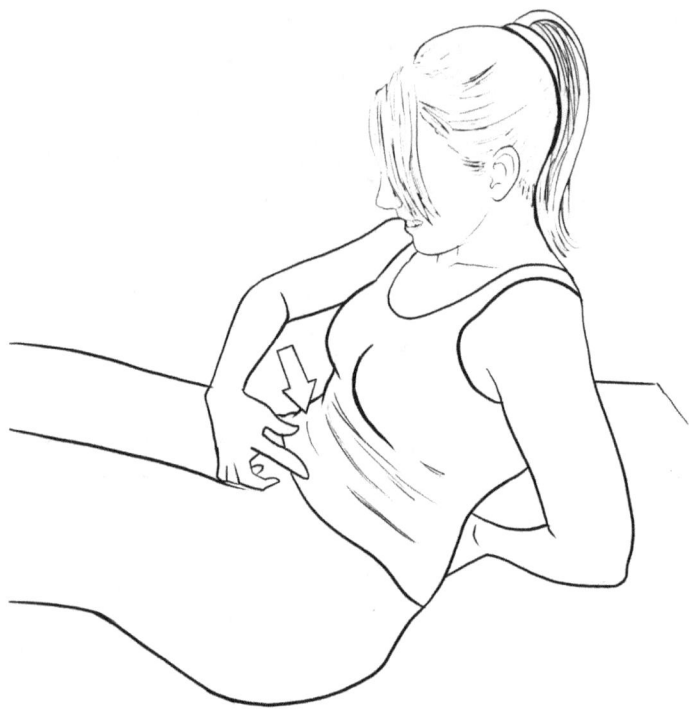

- Sit on the floor with your knees bent in front of you. Hold onto your knees to sit upright.
- Bring hands behind your head for extra support.
- Begin to roll the lowest part of your back toward the floor.
- Continue to roll until you feel your core quiver and shake. Stop there.
- If your neck muscles feel stable enough, extend one arm forward. Relax the head into your other hand.
- Take 3-4 breaths, feeling your core muscles fire.

CHAPTER 7: EXERCISES FOR HEAD AND NECK HEALTH

- If this feels okay, pulse your arm in place for 5 seconds. Then switch the hands and pulse for another 5 seconds.
- Come up, hold onto your knees, lift the chest, and rest.
- Repeat.

*This is a great exercise if you can't sit up from a lying flat position.

#keepingtrack

During this exercise, I felt _____
_____
_____
_____
_____
_____
_____
_____
_____
_____
_____

After this exercise, I felt _____
_____
_____
_____
_____
_____
_____
_____
_____
_____

Crunch
3 reps–1 set/day
with a 30 sec. Rest between sets

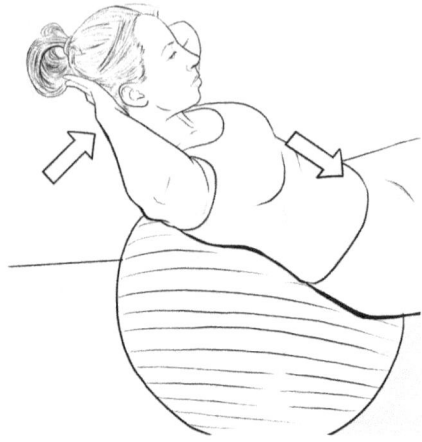

- Option to lie flat on the floor with the knees bent or to sit on an exercise ball. Press your belly button and lower back down toward the floor or ball. Take the hands to the back of the head.
- Lift the upper back, shoulder blades, and head off of the floor or ball—relax the head into your hands, and keep lifting into a crunch.
- Continue to press the lower back down and breathe into your shaking core muscles for three to four breaths.
- Repeat.

#keepingtrack

During this exercise, I felt _____

_____

After this exercise, I felt _____

_____

CHAPTER 7: EXERCISES FOR HEAD AND NECK HEALTH

Foam Roller Crunch
3 reps–1 set/day
with a 30 sec. rest between sets

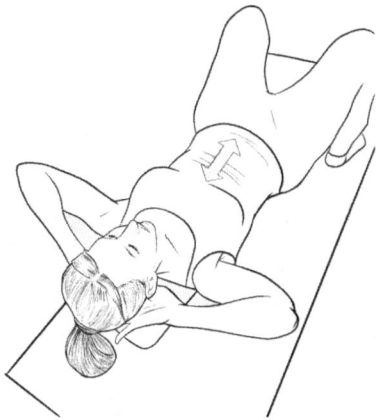

- This is the same as the crunch, with added instability.
- Sit on one side of the roller with your head resting on the other side of the roller.
- Press your belly button down toward the roller and lift into a crunch.
- Again, keep the head and neck relaxed, while lifting the upper back off the roller.

*You need a full length foam roller.

#keepingtrack

During this exercise, I felt _____
_____

After this exercise, I felt _____
_____

Relax with a Foam Roll Under Low Back

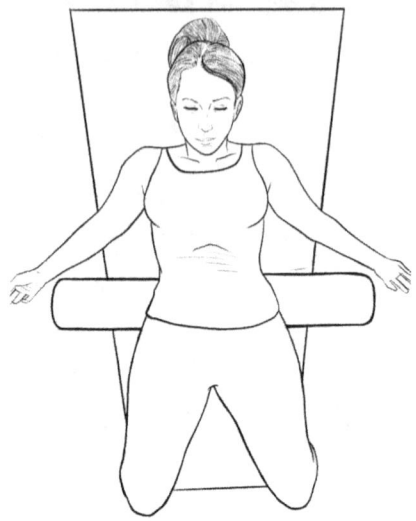

- Lie flat on your back with knees bent.
- Lift hips up and slide the foam roller under your lower back. If this creates too much tension in the neck and shoulders, consider using a half yoga block and gradually increase to the full foam roller.
- Allow the sacrum (the triangular bone at the base of the spine) to rest onto the chosen object and relax.
- This will stretch out your core stomach muscles, open your chest muscles, and relax your shoulder blades.

#*keepingtrack*

During this exercise, I felt _____

_____

After this exercise, I felt _____

_____

CHAPTER 7: EXERCISES FOR HEAD AND NECK HEALTH

*Don't overdo it! Practice only the recommended amount of reps and sets, even if you're feeling ambitious. Also, if you find it difficult to stick with a movement practice in complete silence, find music you enjoy that will motivate you to practice daily.

Create a workout just for you by saying how many reps felt good to practice and keep track below. If you don't think the exercise is helpful, put a line through the rep section for now.

Core Exercises	Reps
Seated Pulsing Abs	
Slow Roll Down	
Crunch	
Foam Roller Crunch	
Relax with Foam Roll Under Low Back	

TWIST EXERCISES

Now that you've woken up your core muscles, you'll be more prepared to safely twist the spine and neck. These twists will also open up the upper back and prepare your body to practice the back extension exercises that are up next. Below you will find three ways to twist and create more movement in the upper spine and neck. Practice one of the poses once a day. I recommend starting with the first pose and moving onto the second one after a week or so.

Windshield Wiper Twist
5 reps on each side—1 set/day

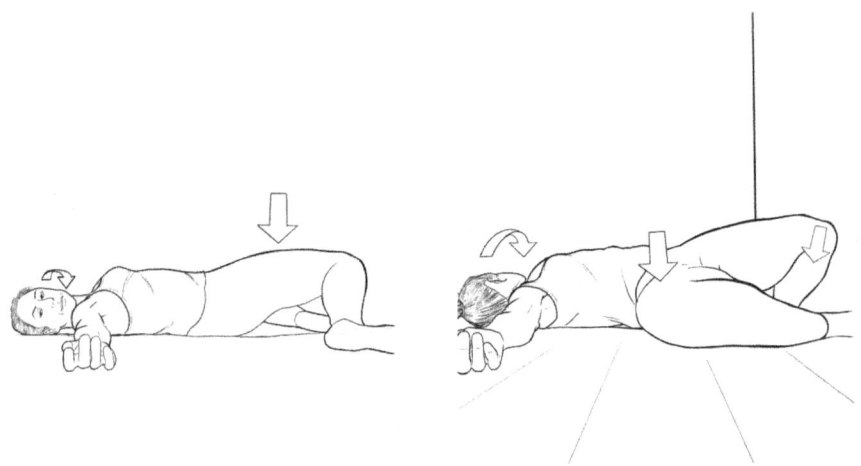

This posture is one of my favorites! It doesn't take a lot of effort, and it can feel amazing.

- Lay flat on your back with your knees bent and feet planted a little wider than hip distance apart. Extend arms out to the sides. Make sure they are in line with your shoulders and not creeping up toward your head. This will keep length in the neck.

CHAPTER 7: EXERCISES FOR HEAD AND NECK HEALTH

- Take a full breath in and feel the length in your spine and neck.
- Exhale. Drop your knees over to the right side and rotate your neck to the left side.
- Inhale. Come back to center, so the knees stack over the hips, and the gaze is focused on the ceiling. Exhale. Drop your knees over to the left side and rotate your head to the right side.
- Inhale. Come back to center.
- On your final repetition, let the knees relax. Take 3-4 breaths in the gentle twist.

*If you experience pain in your neck when you look to the opposite side, then you can either not turn the head as far or turn the head in the same direction as the knees. With practice over time, your range of motion will increase.

#keepingtrack

During this exercise, I felt _____

After this exercise, I felt _____

Simple Standing Twist
5 reps on each side—1 set/day

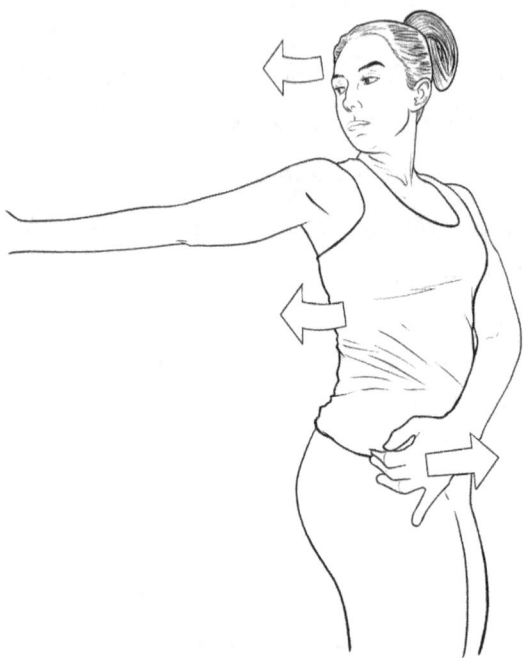

This posture is wonderful because you can do it anywhere. If you're someone who commutes or sits a lot for work, I highly recommend this stretch at least once a day. It will help create mobility in your neck and spine AND give you better posture throughout the day.

- Stand with the feet hip distance apart.
- Inhale and take the arms out to the sides, so they are level with the shoulders. Turn palms forward.
- Exhale and soften the tops of the shoulders, the sides of the neck, and the jaw.
- Inhale and feel the top of your head reach toward the ceiling. Feel all the sides of the neck elongate.

CHAPTER 7: EXERCISES FOR HEAD AND NECK HEALTH

- Exhale and twist to the right. Extend the right arm behind you. Hips are going to want to turn with you; don't let them. Imagine you have headlights on the front of the hips, and those headlights are going to stay pointed straight ahead.

- Inhale. Come back to center with arms stretched out to the sides and the gaze forward. Feel the length through the spine and neck.

- Exhale twist to the left. Extend the left arm behind you. Keep the hips pointed straight ahead. Turn the gaze toward the back arm. Breathe into the upper back, between the shoulder blades, and with each exhale, twist a tiny bit deeper.

- Inhale, return to center, and relax the arms

#keepingtrack

During this exercise, I felt _____
_____
_____
_____
_____
_____
_____
_____

After this exercise, I felt _____
_____
_____
_____
_____
_____
_____

Lunge Twist with the Wall
5 reps on each side—1 set/day

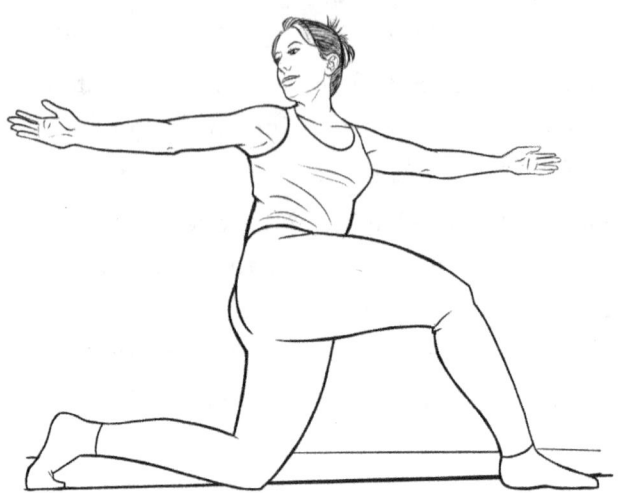

This posture will create more mobility in the upper back and neck. You will need a cushion under your knee, a yoga block, and a wall with nothing around to obstruct movement.

- Take a towel and fold in half, then fold it in half again.
- Stand with the right shoulder facing the wall and step the right leg behind you. Bend the back knee and place the towel underneath it. You will be in a low lunge position.
- Place the yoga block between the wall and the left knee. This will keep the hips aligned, so that you'll get more of a stretch in the upper spine.
- Reach both arms straight ahead. The right arm will stay connected to the wall for the entire exercise, and the left knee will keep the block pressed into the wall.
- Inhale. Open the left arm out to the side and extend it behind you. Take the gaze with you as far as you can without pain.

CHAPTER 7: EXERCISES FOR HEAD AND NECK HEALTH

- Exhale. Bring the left hand forward to meet the right hand and repeat five times on this side.
- Release the block, gently come out of the lunge and turn around so that the left side of your body is facing the wall and the left leg is extended back with the left knee on the towel.
- Place the yoga block between the wall and the right knee.
- Reach the arms straight ahead. The left arm will stay connected to the wall for the entire exercise, and the knee will keep the block pressed into the wall.
- Inhale. Open the right arm out to the side and extend it behind you. Turn the head in the direction of the arm, as far as you can without pain.
- Exhale. Bring the right hand forward to meet the left hand. Repeat 5x on this side.

#*keepingtrack*

During this exercise, I felt _____
_____
_____
_____
_____
_____

After this exercise, I felt _____
_____
_____
_____
_____

Relax with Floor Twist
1-2 minutes

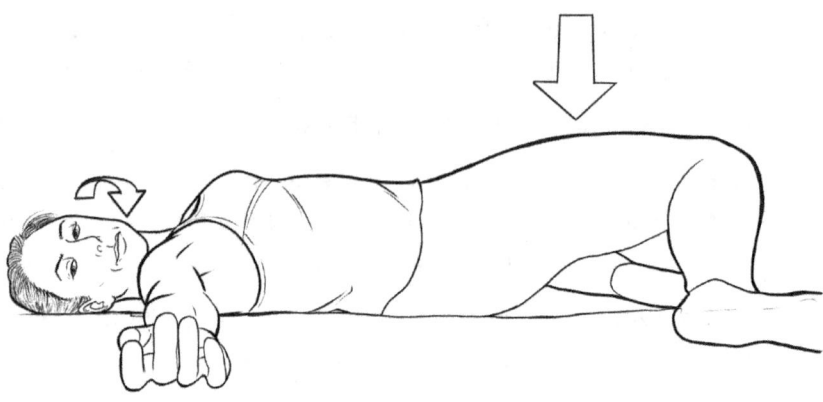

- Come onto the back and extend the arms out to the sides in a T position.
- Bend the knees and lower them to one side.
- Look over the opposite shoulder.
- Rest into this pose. Inhale. Open the right arm out to the side and extend it behind you. Turn the head in the direction of the arm, as far as you can without pain.

*If you'd like more support in this pose you can bring a bolster or some pillows underneath the legs.

#keepingtrack

During this exercise, I felt _____

After this exercise, I felt _____

CHAPTER 7: EXERCISES FOR HEAD AND NECK HEALTH

BACK EXTENSION EXERCISES

Now that you've built core strength and practiced twists to open the upper back, you're ready for these back extension exercises. These poses will stretch your chest and front neck muscles. Practice the dynamic cat/cow pose first, and slowly add in another exercise as your neck feels stronger.

In every back extension posture, you are lengthening the spine. Always think of extending the top of your head toward the ceiling, before arching the back into extension. The goal is to get more movement in the upper portion of the back, not to further compress the back of the neck or the lower back. Don't practice these poses if you've experienced whiplash recently. Give your neck muscles time to recover and then gradually add these in.

Dynamic Cat/Cow
6 reps–1 set/day

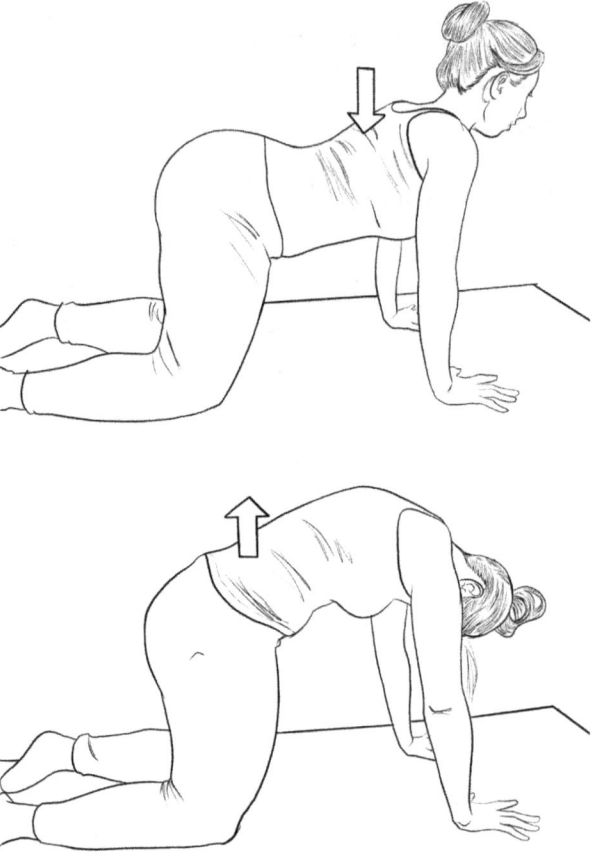

This posture is recommended by physical therapists, chiropractors, yoga instructors, pilates instructors, and that is not a coincidence. It is the simplest way to achieve neck and back extension. This is a dynamic stretch that will create more mobility in your neck and spine.

1. Come onto the hands and knees.
2. Inhale. Let the belly and chest drop toward the floor and lift the gaze forward. Keep length at the back of the neck.

3. Exhale. Push the floor away, let the head drop toward the floor, pull the belly button toward the back and point the tailbone toward the floor.
4. Inhale lower the belly to stretch the front of the torso and lift the head to stretch the front of the throat.
5. Exhale round the back to stretch the back of the neck and entire back.

*Get a free video demonstration with guided instruction of Cat/Cow at https://www.getwellwithdanielle.com/free3dayplan by signing up to receive the free 3 day plan to relieve head and neck pain.

#*keepingtrack*

During this exercise, I felt _____
_____
_____
_____
_____
_____
_____
_____
_____

After this exercise, I felt _____
_____
_____
_____
_____
_____
_____
_____
_____

Back Extension with a Foam Roller
Hold for 3 - 5 breaths

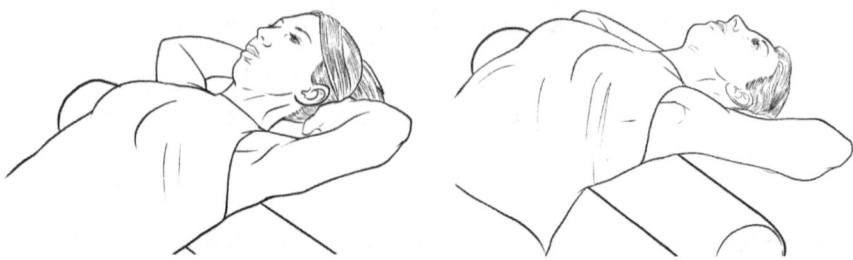

This is a passive stretch, meaning the goal is to relax with little-to-no effort. Let the weight of your head rest into your hands and allow your elbows to drop toward the floor behind you. This will stretch out the front of the neck and the chest muscles.

- Lie with the foam roller across the mid-back, right across the area where a sports bra might be.
- Support the back of the head with hands, and rest the head into extension.
- Go only as far back as it feels good—you can slowly increase with time.

#keepingtrack

During this exercise, I felt _____
_____
_____

After this exercise, I felt _____
_____
_____

Standing Back Extension
Hold for 3 - 5 breaths

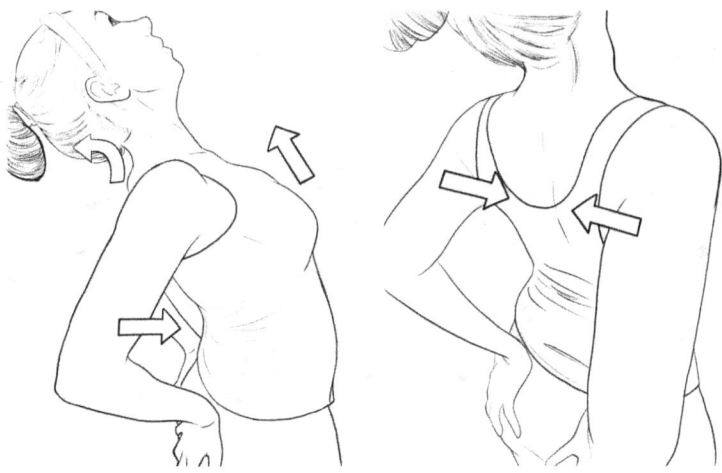

This stretch takes more effort and focus. It's easy to drop the head back and compress the muscles in the back of the neck and head. Don't do that; it won't help your head and neck pain feel better. With each inhale, lengthen through all sides of the neck even as you begin to take the head back into neck extension.

- Stand with feet hip-distance apart.
- Place hands on the lower back and outer hip area with fingers pointing down. Make sure the hands are low enough that the shoulders aren't creeping up toward the ears.
- Draw the elbows toward the back of the room, and feel the muscles between the shoulder blades engage.
- Lift the chest and the gaze until the back and neck are extending backward.
- Go only as far as feels good. Take 3-5 breaths here.

Back Extension on the Floor
5 reps–1 set/day

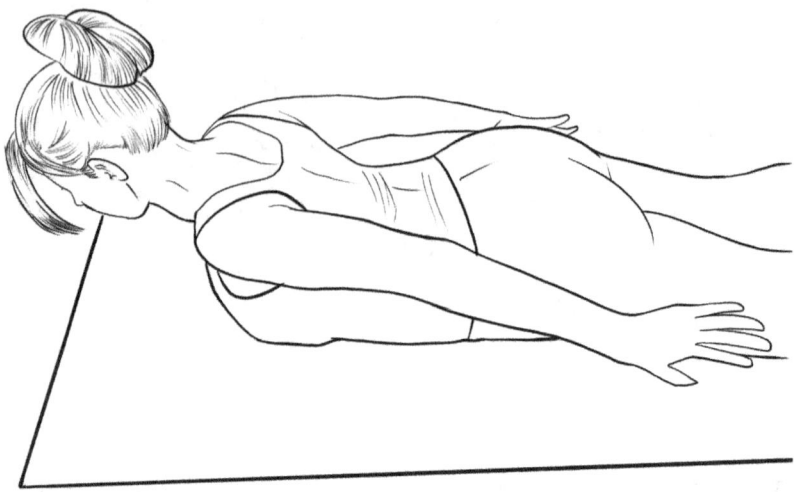

This pose is going to strengthen the muscles that take you into back and neck extension. If you experience pain in the center of the low back or in the back of the neck, try this exercise with a large exercise ball under your belly. Still in pain? Reach out to me at getwellwithdanielle.com

- Lie flat on the stomach and rest the chin or forehead on the floor. Take the arms down to the sides of the body.
- On the inhale, lift head, shoulders, and arms.
- Turn the palms to face inward toward the body.
- Hug the shoulders together and keep length along the sides of the neck.
- Take a full breath here.
- Exhale. Relax the whole body back to the floor.
- Inhale and repeat.

CHAPTER 7: EXERCISES FOR HEAD AND NECK HEALTH

*A couple of other options:

1. Practice cobra with hands placed under the elbows when you lift up. Use very little arm strength and continue to strengthen the back of the neck and back muscles.

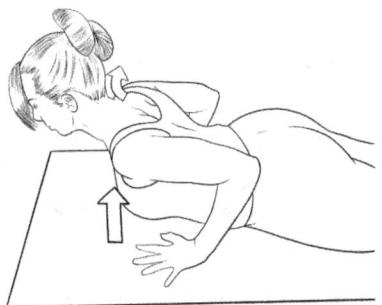

2. This one is more challenging for balance, but can be easier on the lower back. Rest with the belly on an exercise ball. Inhale and lift the head, shoulders, and arms into back extension. Exhale to relax down and rest the hands on the floor.

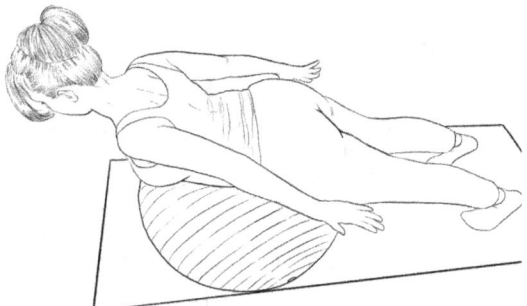

#*keepingtrack*

During this exercise, I felt _____

_____

After this exercise, I felt _____

_____

RELAX with Full Back Extension on an Exercise Ball

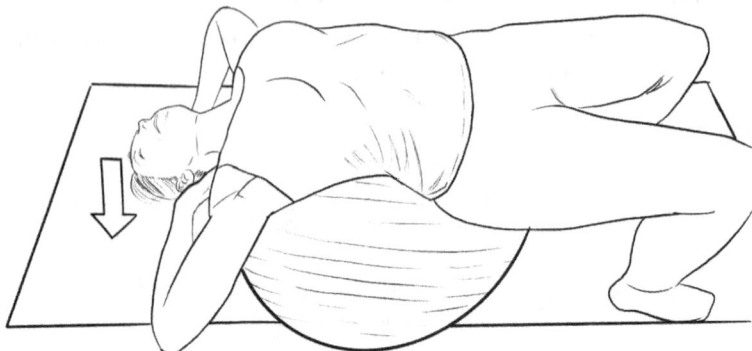

- Lie with the back on a large blow-up exercise ball.
- Support the back of the head with the hands. Lay back so that the head rests on the ball—into extension.
- You can stretch the arms out to the sides in a T position or stretch them overhead.
- Create length in the back of the neck and relax the back of the head onto the ball.
- If you feel low-back or neck pain, don't do this stretch. Instead, return to exercise #1 in the Strengthening Core Exercises before you try this again.

*Remember: Give your body time to heal with these simple exercises. Don't push your body to do too much too fast.

#*keepingtrack*

During this exercise, I felt _____

_____

After this exercise, I felt _____

_____

CHAPTER 7: EXERCISES FOR HEAD AND NECK HEALTH

Create a workout just for you by saying how many reps felt good to practice and keep track below. If you don't think the exercise is helpful, put a line through the rep section for now.

Back Extension Exercises	Reps
Dynamic Cat/Cow	
Back Extension with a Foam Roller	
Standing Back Extension	
Back Extension on the Floor	
Relax with Full Back Extension on an Exercise Ball	

PUT IT ALL TOGETHER

Alright you've made it this far, which means you now have a strong foundation to build upon. You've created a base level of stability, mobility, and strength in the neck, shoulders, spine, core, and now you get to put it all together. The poses below focus on the entire body. After you are comfortable practicing the poses above and below, it's time to add in weight training exercises. I recommend the TRX and resistance bands to begin, then increasing to dumbbell and barbell weight training. If that sounds confusing, find a personal trainer.

Beginning Founder Pose with 3 Arm Variations
3 - 5 breaths, once a day

1. Long Wing Founder

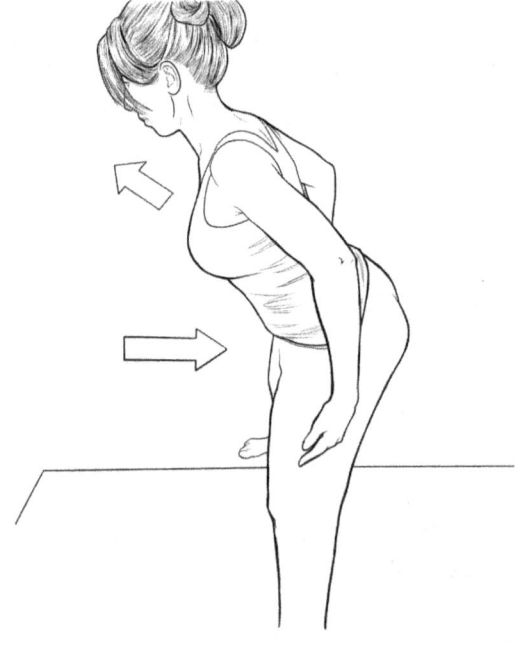

CHAPTER 7: EXERCISES FOR HEAD AND NECK HEALTH

2. Short Wing Founder

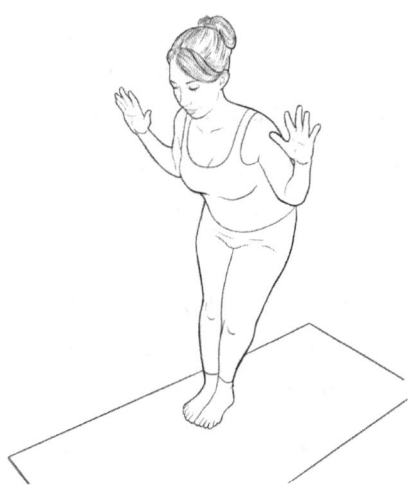

3. Full Founder

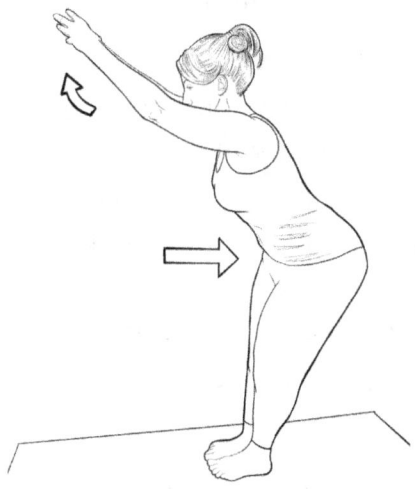

This exercise comes from Foundation Training, and it is one variation of a Founder. You can find wonderful free videos of this exercise at foundationtraining.com, or join my 6 Week Program by going to www.getwellwithdanielle.com/relieveneckpain, where you'll learn more about this pose. Foundation Training also has an incredible streaming platform that goes deep into everything they have to offer.

- Bring the feet hip distance apart with the outer edges of the feet parallel.
- Take arms down to the sides and rotate arms out so the palms face forward. This is called Long Wing position.
- Take a slight bend into the elbows and take a deep breath in. Each time you breathe in, expand the rib cage in every direction.
- Pull the hips back an inch or two, this is called a Hip Hinge. Take the hands forward and bring the finger tips together to create a sphere of tension. Make a ball with the hands and press the tips of the fingers into each other.
- Unlock the knees and pull them behind the heels. If you get the sensation of falling backwards, that's good; it means all of the muscles along the back side of your body are engaging. Push the feet down into the floor. This is called Anchoring the Legs.
- Pull the chin back and the chest up.
- Inhale to expand the entire rib cage, from side to side, front to back, and top to bottom.
- Exhale and contract the entire rib cage. Imagine you are pulling the rib cage off of the lower back. If this doesn't make sense or doesn't feel good, that's okay; just focus on getting the knees behind the heels and keeping the chest up, chin back.
- Repeat for 3-5 breaths.

#*keepingtrack*

During this exercise, I felt _____

_____

After this exercise, I felt _____

_____

Exercise Ball Crunch with Back Extension
5-10 reps–1 set/day
with a 30 sec. rest

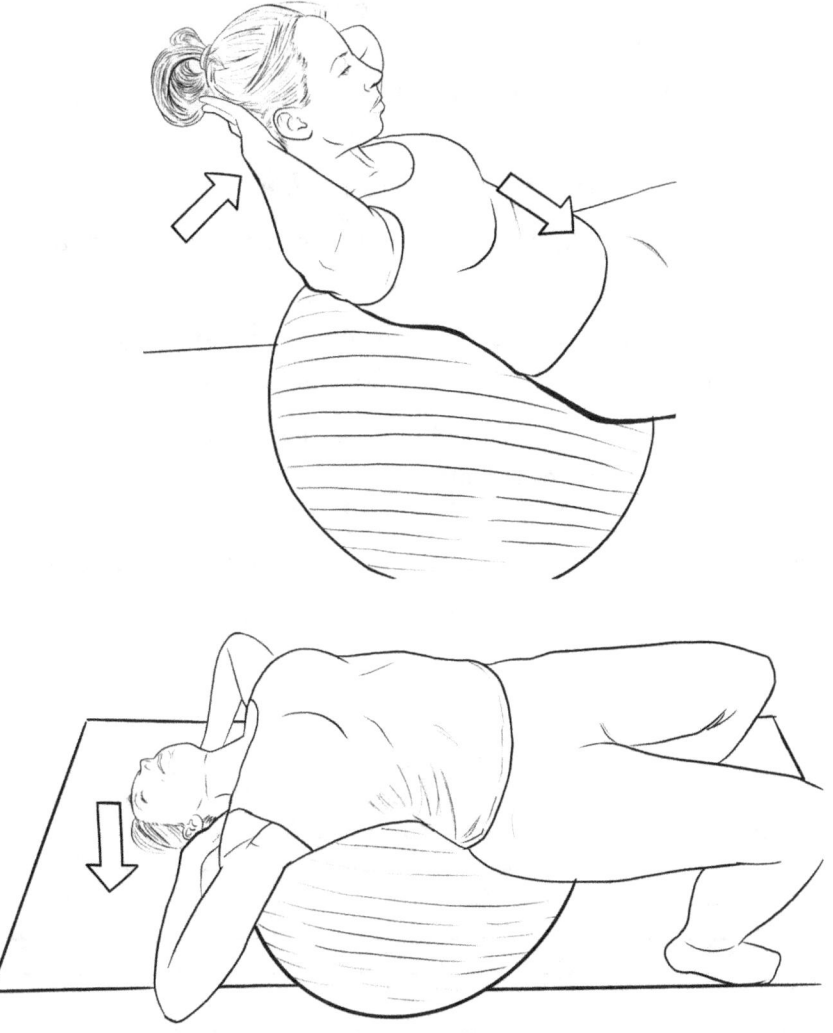

If you develop the needed neck and core strength, then back extension will feel good on the ball, and you can enjoy a nice stretch across the chest and stomach by allowing your head to drop into neck and back extension. If it doesn't feel good, practice the modification below, and try it again at another time.

- Sit on an exercise ball and take hands behind the head.
- Lay back, so the lower and middle back are on the ball. Then take the head back into extension. If you feel a painful pinch in the low back or neck, don't allow the head to drop further than the shoulders.
- On the exhale, add a crunch to strengthen the core.
- Inhale and take the head back into extension as far as feels good.
- Exhale. Lift into a crunch. Think of tightening a belt around the waist as you hold the crunch for 3-5 breaths.
- Over time, use hands behind the head less and less to further strengthen the neck muscles.

*Remember to practice the easier back extension options before this exercise.

#keepingtrack

During this exercise, I felt _____
_____
_____
_____

After this exercise, I felt _____
_____
_____
_____

Forearm Plank
Hold for 30-60 sec.

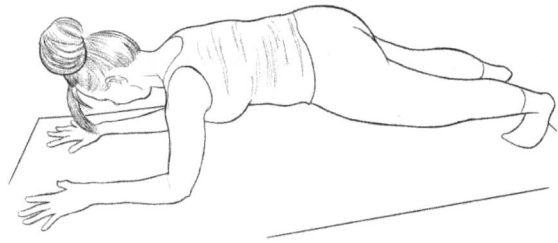

This pose will use all of your muscles. I find it helpful to put on a motivating song when I practice plank; otherwise 30 seconds feels like an eternity!

- Lie on the stomach.
- Place elbows under the shoulders. Flatten forearms and palms on the floor, or interlace the hands and tuck in the pinky fingers.
- Take a breath in, and on the exhale, tuck the toes and lift the knees.
- Inhale and lengthen through all sides of the neck.
- Exhale and firm the thighs up toward the ceiling.
- Keep taking full breaths for 30-60 seconds.

*Option to have someone place a foam roller along the length of the back. Press the back of the head into the roller and draw the belly button up toward the roller. Feel the length of the spine.

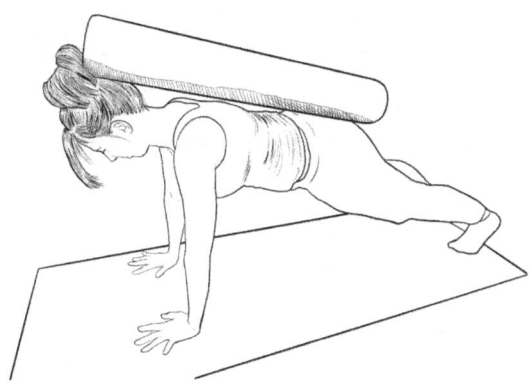

EMPOWERED CHOICES: A GUIDE TO HEALING HEAD & NECK PAIN

Create a workout just for you by saying how many reps felt good to practice and keep track below. If you don't think the exercise is helpful, put a line through the rep section for now.

Putting it All Together Exercises	Reps
Beginning Founder with 3 Arm Variations: 1. Long Wing 2. Short Wing 3. Full Founder	
Exercise Ball Crunch with Back Extension	
Forearm Plank	
Relax with Foam Roll Pec Stretch	

#keepingtrack

During this exercise, I felt _____

_____

After this exercise, I felt _____

_____

CHAPTER 8

FIND A HEALING PROFESSIONAL

I am going to help you navigate the personal training, massage, and yoga world by sharing what to look for when choosing a healing professional. Want a more detailed description of each modality? Check out the detailed resources in chapters 11 and 12.

Do you know where the closest gym, personal trainers, massage therapy, and yoga classes are offered? If not, Google it and read testimonials! Notice if any facility or person stands out to you. It helps if you like the person and the place. The more convenient, the more likely you are to do it. Interested in online training? Flip a few pages ahead to the Online Training section in this chapter.

Some trainers, massage therapists, and yoga instructors will come to your home. If you're pressed for time and can afford this option, ask if they offer this service.

Is there a personal trainer, yoga, pilates, or other instructor you've heard about, but haven't reached out to? Now is the time.

Dealing with an injury and need personal attention, but can't afford an hour of a professional's time? See if the person offers a half hour option, a package, or buddy sessions at a reduced rate. If I know I am going to see someone weekly for a few months or longer, I often extend packages to lower the cost for clients.

WHAT DO I LOOK FOR IN A PERSONAL TRAINER?

Step 1: Be sure that your personal trainer is minimally certified from one of the organizations below. To become a certified personal trainer, most choose from these top 5 certifications. Note: It is not enough for a personal trainer to be certified. Make sure they have continuing education and certifications. Ex: TRX certification, Foundation Training certification, or other proof of study as a coach.

- NASM (National Academy of Sport Medicine)
- ISSA (International Sports Sciences Association)
- ACE (American Council on Exercise
- ACSM (American College of Sports Medicine)
- NSCA (National Strength and Conditioning Association)

Double check your trainers certification at the sites above. https://www.nasm.org/resources/validate-credentials will take you to a place to verify my certification.

Step. 2: Once you've verified the above, review the trainer's testimonials, reviews, or website.

Step 3: Satisfied? If so, reach out. Ask them to explain their philosophy and the goals they help clients reach.

It is important to find a trainer who will help you reach your goals. Examples:

- If you want to run a marathon and have never run before, find a trainer who specializes in marathon running.
- If you're going to run a marathon and you're already an incredible runner, but you keep injuring yourself because you lack mobility and flexibility, find a trainer who specializes in assisted stretching, flexibility, or Foundation Training. FoundationTraining.com offers an incredible resource to find a trainer near you. When you click on the instructor, it shows their level of Foundation Training certification and their modalities.

Step 4: Does it sound and feel like a good fit? If so, book a trial session!

HOW DO I FIND A MASSAGE OR CRANIOSACRAL THERAPIST?

Many Chiropractors work with massage therapists, so this is a great first place to check. You can go to a spa and if you happen to fall in love with a massage therapist, ask if you can book regularly with them or if they work outside of the spa. Many therapists have other jobs or offer massages in other locations.

When looking for an independent massage therapist or CranioSacral therapist, a quick GoogleMaps search will bring up people near you. Be sure they have a state massage therapy certification. Most are practicing legally, but it's important to make sure. Especially if you're going into someone's home for a massage.

Most states require extensive training, although some cities have lower standards, or people working illegally. For example, there was a time when someone could practice massage in San Francisco with only 100 hours of massage training, and in Oakland 300 hours of training was sufficient. Not sure what your state requirements are? Find out here: https://www.abmp.com/practitioners/state-requirements

My favorite way to find a new therapist is to ask around. Most people are happy to share resources and are likely to send you to someone who can help alleviate your pain. This is especially true when searching for a CranioSacral Therapist.

Massage therapists are not the only practitioners who offer CranioSacral therapy; many chiropractors, orthopedic doctors, and some physical therapists offer it as well.

HOW DO I FIND A YOGA TEACHER?

Yoga instructors can be found in yoga studios, gyms, and online. Most studios require teachers to complete a 200 hour yoga certification; others ask for 500 hours. Many studios want instructors to be certified in their brand of yoga, which is unfortunate for yoga instructors who already have 500 hours of training with no interest in paying for another 200 hour training.

Many incredible teachers can be found at your local gym. However, in some gyms it is sufficient to teach yoga with a trendy choreographed yoga certification. These kinds of certifications, such as BodyFlow and Buti yoga, can be acquired in a weekend. They cram the instructors with information, choreography, music, and then they have to prove they are capable of teaching the material. It's important for you to know if your yoga teacher has received a basic 200 hour or 500 hour yoga training before taking the trendy yoga certification. If it's your first time attending a yoga class and you're in a BodyFlow or Buti Yoga class, know that these classes tend to be fun, fast paced, and challenging for people who are already in shape. Be sure to take the modifications and go at your pace.

If you seek a yoga instructor to work privately with an injury, make sure they have a 500 hour certification, previous training working with injuries, a massage background, or another equivalent training that gives them the tools to work with you. Ideally, they will also have a yoga therapy certification, Iyengar certification, a Pilates background or some equal in-depth training to help treat your injury. Many incredible systems exist; just confirm that the source of their education appeals to you.

A Word of Warning: Beware of cheap fitness courses that cram in information without teaching trainers how to build stability and how to pursue rehab in a safe way. Make sure the person you are working with is qualified to help you. If you're already taking yoga classes from an instructor you love who is helping you get stronger, more flexible, and feel better, but your injury keeps being aggravated, ask if they offer private sessions. Yoga was originally taught one-on-one and, although teachers do their best to address all body types in a class, it's impossible to teach directly to each person's needs. Even one private session will benefit your overall practice.

ONLINE TRAINING

If you live in an area where in-person classes aren't available and you can't find trainers near you, consider online options. The pandemic shifted many offerings online or hybrid, so you can access incredible instructors from all over the world.

The benefits of online training is that you can practice in the comfort of your home, for just a few minutes each day or longer, and it can be more cost effective. The downside is you won't get to practice face-to-face with someone, so they can't offer hands-on adjustments, although this might be an upside to some people. Ask yourself what you need, and reach for it!

Sites to help you find personal trainers and yoga instructors online or in-person:

- Get Well with Danielle: https://www.getwellwithdanielle.com/1-1-sessions
- Foundation Training: https://www.foundationtraining.com/find-a-foundation-trainer/
- IdeaFit: https://pro.ideafit.com/find-personal-trainer
- YogaWorks: https://www.yogaworks.com (an incredible place for beginners to start with instructors who have been well trained)
- Yoga Nidra or Therapeutic Yoga: Check out my group classes for online offerings at www.getwellwithdanielle.com/group-sessions (These will help if you have chronic pain or need help managing your stress level.)

If you're not interested in yoga or personal training, but still want to learn to move your body in new ways, look up YouTube videos that show you how to isolate movements. This will help you get into your body, feel into your hips, shoulders, and just get moving. In college, I had the comical experience of trying a belly dance class, and, when I attempted to move my body parts separately from one another, it was laughable. Moving my shoulder without moving my torso was not an option. To me, they were one and the same; I didn't think it was possible to move them as separate entities. The practice of isolating parts helped connect me to new muscles, and doing this practice in the privacy of my home was necessary :)

CHAPTER 8: FIND A HEALING PROFESSIONAL

MIND STILL TRICKING YOU WITH UNHELPFUL THOUGHTS?

Use these New Thoughts...

Unhelpful Thoughts	New Thoughts
I don't know who to see.	I'll ask around, do a Google search, and read Yelp reviews.
I don't have the money.	I'll find a local school that offers discounted massages for students to practice, or I'll look for a deal. I'll cut back on everything and save at least $3 a day, so I'll have enough for a massage by the end of the month. It's worth it.
I don't want to take my clothes off and have a stranger massage my body with oil.	I'll look up a type of massage that doesn't require clothes off, such as Thai, Sports, Shiatsu, Acupressure, or CranioSacral.
I don't have the time.	I will make the time because, if my physical well being is compromised, I'm no use to anyone, including myself!
I don't deserve a massage.	It's not about deserving. My body needs maintenance the same way a car or a house needs maintenance. It will function better when properly maintained.

Unhelpful Thoughts	New Thoughts
I'm too busy to work out, and I flake out on what I say I'll do.	I will hire a personal trainer who I can see weekly or biweekly and have regular apportionments. This will hold me accountable to show up.
I hate working out alone.	I can get a buddy to work out with me.
I have injuries and I don't know where to start.	I will find someone with extensive training in Iyengar Yoga, Viniyoga, Restorative yoga, Yoga Therapeutics, Feldenkrais, Pilates, or Foundation Training who can provide personal instruction.
Working out sucks, I know I need to, but I hate the gym.	I can find a fun way to move my body by trying out a dance class, playing with a hula-hoop, jump roping, or going skating.
It is what it is, everyone has pain, I can suck it up and deal with it.	I will get support and age with grace. I can feel-better with more mobility, flexibility, and strength.
I know I need to _____, but _____.	I will take one step toward what I need to do today. No more procrastinating.

CHAPTER 8: FIND A HEALING PROFESSIONAL

THE FIRST 3 SESSIONS!

Now that you've chosen a healing professional, it's time for your first session! When working with any trainer, massage therapist, or yoga instructor, it's important to ask yourself the questions below. This exercise will help you continue making empowered choices that ultimately help you feel good. Circle Yes/No.

Do I trust them?	❑ Yes	❑ No
Did they ask about my previous injuries?	❑ Yes	❑ No
Do they listen to where I have pain?	❑ Yes	❑ No
Do they care about my goals?	❑ Yes	❑ No
Do I feel I'm getting stronger?	❑ Yes	❑ No
Do I feel I'm getting more flexible?	❑ Yes	❑ No
Is my balance improving?	❑ Yes	❑ No
Is the range of motion in my joints increasing?	❑ Yes	❑ No
Are my personal goals being met?	❑ Yes	❑ No
Do I feel empowered working with them?	❑ Yes	❑ No
Do they check in to make sure the methods they are using are helpful?	❑ Yes	❑ No

Answering these questions will help you evaluate. If the answers are a resounding "Yes!" Wonderful! If not, consider how you might ask them to adjust or find a different healing professional. Keep in mind that it can take at least three sessions to get to know someone and for them to get to know you.

For a more specific lens, here are the questions I ask when working with a new client:

- What kind of work do you do?
- What kind of exercise do you do?

- How busy are you?
- What is your stress level?
- Do you have any injuries you're working with?
- What are your immediate goals?
- How can I help?

Most importantly, I listen to what they tell me. On the basis of their answers, we come up with a plan. Together, we decide how much physical activity, relaxation, and stretching to include.

After a few sessions, we may adjust the plan. I usually let the client guide where we go, unless I'm certain they need a gentle push in another direction to reach their goal. I nudge them toward options that I think will benefit them most, but ultimately it's their body and their choice. They decide how often they want to work together, and I accommodate as best I can. Make sure your healing professional shows a genuine interest in learning from you as you progress in sessions and that they pay attention to alignment and safety; especially in the beginning, it's best to get a solid foundation and not hurt yourself.

Everyone has their own style of training, and it's important you enjoy working with them. If someone talks down to you, criticizes you, is harsh with you, and you don't like it, it's not a good fit. If someone makes you feel weak and tells you to "toughen up, and you just feel like they are beating you up week after week, it's not a good fit. If someone doesn't listen to you and isn't working to support your goals, it's not a good fit. Find someone who empowers you to feel better about yourself and stronger in your body.

Keep in mind it takes at least three sessions to get to know someone and for them to get to know you. After you've tried three sessions, you might come across a few problems and need solutions.

CHAPTER 8: FIND A HEALING PROFESSIONAL

PROBLEMS AND SOLUTIONS

Problems	Solutions
I received a massage and it hurt.	I will find someone who practices a modality with a light-touch, such as CranioSacral therapy or light touch Swedish massage. I won't keep going to someone who hurts me.
Every time I work out I hurt myself.	I will find someone who can train me slowly and show me how to not hurt myself.
I didn't feel any benefits from the massage, I barely even felt the massage.	I will find someone who practices with a deeper-touch. Maybe I'll look for someone who specializes in Rolfing or Deep Tissue.
I feel weak after working with a personal trainer who always talks down to me.	I will find a trainer who is encouraging, qualified, and confident in their ability to help me, not cocky and superior, but secure and compassionate. They will listen to me and explain what it is we are doing. Ultimately, it is my body, and I know what is best.
I really like the new person I am working with, but they don't challenge me enough.	I will tell my coach I am ready for more of a challenge, and if after a few sessions, they haven't adjusted the routine, I will find a different person to work with.

CHAPTER 9

EMPOWERED CHOICES FOR SPECIFIC NECK PAIN

This chapter will guide you toward where to begin your practice with the exercises for head and neck health. If you've had a recent concussion, whiplash, or are suffering with depression, read the beginning chapters before diving into the options below. If you're dealing with neck pain that's coming from being on a computer or phone too much, from having a labor intensive job, from being a new mom, from an old injury, from repetitive stress, from having a stiff neck, or from a combination of these, find recommendations to relieve your neck pain below.

CONCUSSIONS AND NECK PAIN

Here's what's up:
A concussion is when you have a forceful blow to the head. There are mild concussions and more severe traumatic brain injury concussions.

According to the CDC, these are 5 signs of a concussion:

- Headache or "pressure" in head.
- Nausea or vomiting.
- Balance problems or dizziness, or double or blurry vision.
- Bothered by light or noise.
- Feeling sluggish, hazy, foggy, or groggy.
- Confusion, concentration, or memory problems.
- Not "feeling right" or "feeling down".

The CDC's "danger signs" to look out for after a concussion:

- One pupil is larger than the other.
- Drowsiness or inability to wake up.
- A headache that gets worse and does not go away.
- Slurred speech, weakness, numbness, or decreased coordination.
- Repeated vomiting or nausea, convulsions or seizures (shaking or twitching).
- Unusual behavior, increased confusion, restlessness, or agitation.
- Loss of consciousness (passed out/knocked out). Even a brief loss of consciousness should be taken seriously.

It's important to see a doctor to determine how bad your concussion is and then find the appropriate healing program for you.

Here's what I recommend:

- Stay away from too much screen time, bright lights, and sounds for a few days, maybe longer, depending on how you feel.
- Rest. You suffered an injury and need time to heal.
- Don't sleep too much, even though you might want to sleep a lot, you don't need more sleep than you usually, that's just your concussion talking.

- Listen to your body and take it easy, but don't stop all activity.
- Take a short walk.
- Get your blood circulating.
- Do a short meditation focused on a simple breathing exercise to increase your overall well being.
- Eventually, receive CranioSacral Therapy. It will help you let go of stored tension in your body.
- If short walks lead to feeling nauseous, dizzy, or out of breath, take it easy before you increase.
- Be kind to yourself. Just because you can't see the injury doesn't mean you aren't injured.
- Give yourself time to heal and know that it may take longer than 2-6 weeks, especially if you push yourself.

WHIPLASH AND NECK PAIN

Here's what's up:

Whiplash is when your head whips forward or backward past a normal range of motion into hyperextension and hyperflexion. When this happens, it's possible to injure your neck muscles, tendons, ligaments, your spine or the discs between your spine. Whiplash can cause tension headaches that usually start at the base of the skull and neck pain that you feel in the front or back of the neck. After whiplash, it can hurt to move your head in any or all directions.

If you never received treatment for whiplash, it may have led to chronic neck pain that persists for years. That's what happened to my neck.

Here's what I recommend:
- Work individually with a trained and skilled yoga therapist, physical therapist, or chiropractor. Preferably someone who offers movement and massage.
- If you don't feel improvement after a month or two, switch to a different practitioner. I know it can be time consuming and exhausting to find someone new, but sometimes it's necessary to get the right kind of care for yourself.

DEPRESSION AND NECK PAIN

Here's what's up:
You may have depression for a multitude of reasons. Maybe it's coming from an old traumatic brain injury or other injury, maybe it's coming from having chronic neck pain, maybe it's coming from living in a human body, being overly empathetic, and not knowing how to deal with all the suffering in the world, and maybe it's coming from all of this and more. Whatever the reason, it's important to acknowledge that you feel persistent sadness, despair, and loneliness.

Here's what I recommend:
- If your depression is leading to suicidal thoughts, call the Suicide & Crisis Lifeline @ 988 or the National Suicide Prevention Hotline @ (800) 273-8255. They are available 24/7.
- You're not alone in feeling the way you feel, even though it may feel that way.
- Meditate on visualizations that make you feel better. See yourself in a situation that is supportive and loving. Make a vision board and imagine that your life exists inside of the images. Or create a journal and slowly fill it with joyous, open-hearted, and fun experiences.

CHAPTER 9: EMPOWERED CHOICES FOR SPECIFIC NECK PAIN

- Listen to motivational or inspiring meditations to get your mind set on a new pathway.
- Practice loving-kindness toward yourself and extend it out toward others.
- Repeat the mantra, "I exist therefore I matter."
- Stay away from people who cause you harm or who use you as their dumping ground. Protect yourself.
- Write a lot. Write out all of your thoughts. Write letters to anyone who has caused you harm or to the parts of yourself that cause you harm and then write letters to kindness and love, asking them to guide you.
- Write a letter to yourself, but start with Dear friend, and then tell yourself your problem and respond the way a friend would respond. This exercise comes from *"Fierce Compassion"* by Kristen Neff, Ph.D. A kind, loving, compassionate, take no bull shit kind-of-friend. If it helps, put the letter up where you can see it.
- Seek therapy. Cognitive behavioral therapy is especially helpful when dealing with depression.

"TECH" OR "TEXT" NECK PAIN

Here's what's up:
Your neck muscles are getting tight from being in one position all day. You probably have a combination of forward head posture and chronically looking down posture. The nerves at the base of the spine are likely being compressed, your front neck muscles are overly tight, and if you're stressed out your shoulders are probably elevated, which is all adding to your stiff tech or text neck pain after a long day of 8-10+ hours on the phone or computer.

Here's what I recommend:

- First, practice the isometric contraction exercises.
- Then practice the restorative back extension exercises.
- Work your way up to the harder back extension exercises in combination with the core exercises. This is the best general place to start building back your neck strength and correcting your posture.

LABOR INTENSIVE NECK PAIN

Here's what's up:

If you're a mechanic, a construction worker, or someone who does labor intensive work, your muscles are tight and stiff. If you don't receive regular massages at least every couple of months then your neck is going to be tight often. It's possible when you go to work out it will add to your already tight neck muscles.

Here's what I recommend:

Seek a deep tissue, sports, or deep Swedish massage every other month or minimally twice a year, and practice these self-massage techniques below:

- Use the S-curve self-massager to pin and stretch your muscles.
- Use the foam roller to roll out your upper back and to relax your head into back extension.
- You can find a short video about how to use these on my blog at getwellwithdanielle.com/blog

CHAPTER 9: EMPOWERED CHOICES FOR SPECIFIC NECK PAIN

NEW MAMA NECK PAIN

Here's what's up:

You're most likely spending everyday looking down at your adorable creation. Maybe you're feeding a new baby and carrying it all day everyday or you're chasing around and holding your active toddler all day. Either way, your neck is doing so much work. You might have neck spasms, cramps, headaches that are coming from neck pain, or an overall stiff neck. You might also have neck pain that's coming from not caring for yourself and not having the time to do the things you love.

Here's what I recommend:

- If you've got a new baby you're caring for, make sure your arms are propped up with pillows when you're feeding the baby so that your neck can relax.

- Practice looking straight ahead or up toward the ceiling when you can to keep your head and neck from getting locked up.

- Practice one of the neck extension exercises. Find the one that feels good in your body and do it everyday. It will help relieve your neck pain, by doing the opposite of what it is you're doing all day.

- If you have time for a massage, do it! If not, practice one of the pin and stretch self-massage techniques, or find something that sounds inviting from the feel-good chapter tips.

- Carve out a small window of time each day to do something for yourself that doesn't involve laundry, diapers, or feedings.

OLD INJURIES AND NECK PAIN

Here's what's up:
Maybe you never took the time to heal an old injury. Maybe you started doing a new movement practice and now the old pain has returned. Maybe someone told you, or you told yourself, you have to learn to live with the neck pain you've had ever since the old injury. Maybe there's an emotional and physical block that your body is carrying around from your old injury. Maybe it never healed right and needs physical therapy. One way or the other, the pain has returned to teach you something. Do your best to stay open to the wisdom of your body and take daily steps to heal.

Here's what I recommend:

- Write about where you think the pain is coming from.
- Schedule a massage, CranioSacral Therapy, or any other therapeutic hands on touch modality to help your nervous system relax and let go of the trauma stored in your body from the old injury.
- Find one strengthening exercise and one relaxation exercise in this book that feels good to practice. Add it to your daily self-care. You can start with the first exercise in each section and work your way up to practicing more exercises.
- If you don't notice progress, book a session with a trained movement specialist. You can find more detailed ways to do that in the Finding a Healing Professional section.

REPETITIVE STRESS AND NECK PAIN

Here's what's up:
You're doing some kind of motion during each day that is aggravating your current neck pain. The first step is to figure out what it is that you're doing that's hurting you. Too much computer time? If so, look up at the "Tech" or "Text" neck pain. Too much tennis, golf, yoga?

Here's an example for you: I used to handwrite in all of my journals for a minimum of ten minutes a day, which was usually more like thirty minutes to an hour a day. When I wrote, I was usually hunched over a table with my right shoulder up around my ear. I had no idea that this was setting off my neck pain until a chiropractor helped point it out. Then I started writing in bed. I laid on my side with a pillow under my head and my elbow propped up on a pillow, my arm and shoulder relaxed, which stopped aggravating my chronic neck pain.

Here's what I recommend:

- Notice the most repetitive movements you do throughout the day and if you have time, write them down.

- Then notice how you feel after you've done those movements. Does it aggravate your neck pain?

- If possible, take a two week break from the repetitive motion and see if that helps. If the pain returns when you go back to the movement, seek a professional to help strengthen the necessary muscles to keep it from happening again.

- Find someone who specializes in healing head and neck pain. Not sure where to start? Go back to the Finding a Healing Professional chapter and find someone who can help.

STIFF NECK PAIN

Here's what's up:

You've been living in your body all these years and accumulating neck tension. Now, you've become aware of how stiff and inflexible your neck has become. You may have grown accustomed to turning your entire body to see what's behind you when you're driving and have to back up. Or maybe you started taking a yoga class and noticed your head barely moves when it comes time to stretch out your neck muscles. If you've got a stiff neck, it's difficult to turn the head side to side, look down or up, and bring your ear toward your shoulder on either side.

Here's what I recommend:

- Work on creating mobility in your neck by following the neck exercises in this book.
- Do this in combination with the pin and stretch self-massage techniques or with the help of a certified massage therapist.

CHAPTER 10

BEFORE YOU GO

Remember to be patient with yourself. Everything in life is impermanent; it is always changing. Even if that change is minuscule and you barely notice it, it's still happening. It might take years or decades, but if you stick with creating new movement habits, no matter how long it takes you to get comfortable, you will be continuously progressing.

Movement can feel good even when it is challenging. If it feels horrible, you're sore all the time, and you don't understand why, then it's equally beneficial to have manual work done and seek a body therapist.

Massage can help you stay off of prescription substances, such as pain meds, alcohol, marijuana, and others. It will give you relief from constant pain. It can release scar tissue that forms from accumulated injuries. It can help you relax and de-stress. You can find all of the massage modalities mentioned at the end of this book under Massage Resources.

CranioSacral therapy alleviates the pressure in the skull from concussions and creates space in the back of the head where muscles may be chronically tight from whiplash. It helps release restrictions that come from traumatic injuries. It allows the body to drop into a deep state of relaxation so that the fascial tissues can unwind.

You don't necessarily need someone to dig into your muscles to get rid of pain. Light-touch modalities can have longer-lasting results. The same is true in reverse: if you're seeking light touch with minimal results, try a technique with more pressure from someone you trust.

After a severe injury, the affected area gets tight, and the nervous system goes into a holding pattern. One way to help your nervous system relax is to practice Savasana. In the practice of yoga, each class ends with Savasana, the final pose where you rest on your back in stillness. All layers of tension begin to melt away as you lie still for 5-10 minutes. Check out YogaNidra and you'll practice deep relaxation for 30 minutes to an hour.

Finally, remember that old saying, "If you don't use it, you lose it." You've been given this body and this injury, and you can't change that, but what are you going to do about it? Drugs and pills won't fix weak muscles. Get up, move more, and do what you can to feel better. Let's teach the next generation that we need to prioritize movement and mental health.

It can help to figure out Your Why. *Why* do you want to heal your head and neck pain? *Why* do you want to practice movement? *Why* does it matter if you can hold a plank or do a sit-up?

For a long time I didn't know what My Why was, but it was inside of me driving my daily choices. I wanted to get out of pain and I didn't want to be overweight, but most of the things I did to work-out hurt. I knew I wanted to be more active, to be able to climb stairs and hike trails without getting winded. I also wanted to have a strong yoga practice because it looked satisfying.

Eventually, I realized My Deeper Why. I wanted to age with grace. I saw three of my great-grandparents live into old age, and their last five years were spent confined to a bed or chair. My great grandma had crippling osteoporosis. None of my grandparents stretched. They gave up walking because they didn't have the energy. Their bodies were broken down from years of hard work. The only reason they continued to survive was because someone else was taking care of them, not to mention their genetics.

Then one day I saw a woman in her late 80's on a talk show, and she was the opposite of my grandparents; she was walking on a tightrope! That's why I get on my yoga mat daily. I want to be like that lady when I grow to be her age.

We all have a unique fitness journey, and yours will be exactly what you need it to be. Keep finding your way and seeking out people who encourage you to move out of problems and into solutions. Your healing puzzle pieces are out there.

Lastly, be gentle with yourself. Remember it takes time to heal, nothing is perfect, but it can get better. Don't let the pain stop you from living a healthier lifestyle. Keep going, one step at a time! That's all any of us can do.

CHAPTER 11

MASSAGE RESOURCES

Find someone in your area who has training in the massage technique you are most interested in or who you've heard has had positive results working with your specific injury. Many massage therapists combine techniques, so if you do or don't want something during your massage, be sure to voice that. It's also important to let your therapist know the kind of pressure you'd like to receive, and to let them know if it's too deep or too light, especially during the first massage. For example, if you're someone who loves or hates your feet being massaged, tell them. It will help you relax deeper during the massage. Types of massage I recommend:

ACUPRESSURE

Don't be fooled: there is no pressure used in this technique. It is a light-touch massage where the therapist holds various points along the meridians. The meridians were once described to me as multiple rivers that distribute chi, or life force energy, throughout the body. When a river isn't flowing properly, it gets blocked, and when the chi can't flow, we experience constricted areas of tension. This works best with energetic restrictions. If you aren't expecting deep touch, then this can be a very relaxing massage. It's amazing the emotional stress you feel melt away as a seasoned practitioner works along the meridians. It's powerful. This modality is traditionally done with clothes on, although some people include it in an oil massage. I love the neck and shoulder release points from Acupressure and include them in almost every massage I give whether the client is clothed or not.

CRANIOSACRAL THERAPY

CranioSacral is based on scientific methods and was created by an Osteopathic doctor. Before the 1920's, it was believed that the bones of the skull were fused in adults. In the 1940s, Dr. William Sutherland, the father of CranioSacral, ran experiments on himself where he'd constrict the bones of his skull and take notes on any changes in his behavior. His wife helped him document these experiments.

It's said that he nearly lost consciousness in his first experiment, and his wife had to help him release the pressure of the helmet he was using. He discovered that, when the contraption was released, there was a fluid movement down his spine and into the sacrum, the big triangular bone at the base of the spine. He continued his experiments and found the same results. This backed his conclusion that the cranial bones and the sacrum moved as a result of the connection in the fascia and connective tissues: the tendons, the ligaments, and the fascia.

CranioSacral Therapy is a light-touch healing modality that aims to release myofascial restrictions. It is performed with clothes on and is sometimes included during an oil massage. Energy work is involved, and it is very much about listening to the client's body and feeling where movement, such as blood flow, cerebral spinal fluid, and softening of muscle tissue, is happening.

CHAPTER 11: MASSAGE RESOURCES

There are two popular ways to practice CranioSacral Therapy: Biodynamic and Biomechanic. Both modalities require a similar pressure applied, which is about the weight of a nickel. It's not a forceful touch, but it can have profound lasting effects. Specifically, it can relax the nervous system, anxiety, and stress, as well as relieve chronic muscular pain, post-traumatic stress disorder, migraines, TMJ dysfunction (jaw deviation), myofascial restrictions, and insomnia.

The Upledger Institute International has been teaching Biomechanical CranioSacral Therapy for many years. According to this well-respected institute, "CranioSacral Therapy (CST) is a gentle, hands-on method of evaluating and enhancing the functioning of a physiological body system called the CranioSacral system comprised of the membranes and cerebrospinal fluid that surround and protect the brain and spinal cord. Using a soft touch (generally no greater than 5 grams or about the weight of a nickel), practitioners release restrictions in the CranioSacral system, which has been shown to improve the functioning of the central nervous system, as well as many other systems of the body, such as digestive, musculoskeletal, respiratory, circulatory, and more. CST has also been shown to help with the physical components related to such somatic conditions as Post Traumatic Stress, depression and anxiety." https://www.upledger.com/therapies/

The Biodynamic approach to CranioSacral Therapy teaches the practitioner to create space and learn to listen to the the natural health in a clients body:

"BCST is a healing art that works with the energies that create and maintain health in the human system. While not a manipulative therapy, it has roots in osteopathy and has evolved to include influences from human development, pre and perinatal psychology, trauma resolution, and recent advances in neuroscience. BCST supports nervous system regulation and allows the resolution of conditions resulting from stress and trauma. Practitioners use an educated, gentle, non-invasive touch to engage with the expressions of health in the system." For more, check out: https://www.CranioSacraltherapy.org/

The main difference from Biomechanic and Biodynamic is that the mechanic comes at it from more of an adjustment side and is manipulating bone movement; the dynamic practitioner is holding space and allowing the body to unwind on its own. I was trained by instructors who practice both ways. In my practice, I move back and forth between these techniques. Here's an article that talks further about the differences between Biodynamic and Biomechanical CranioSacral Therapy: https://www.lumennatura.com/2011/12/15/biomechanical-versus-biodynamic-CranioSacral-therapy/

People who are trained in one modality or the other usually undertake a lot of training in that field. Make sure it's a system that works for you. They are received quite differently and have varying results.

A few of the holds you will experience from a therapist during a CranioSacral session are:

- Hands under the heels of the feet or on top of the feet, having one hand under the sacrum and one above it on the lower belly
- One hand underneath the rib cage and one above it
- One hand underneath the shoulder blades or upper back and one over the chest and heart center
- One hand under the skull and one over the forehead
- One hand under the sacrum and one under the skull

During a one hour session, you may experience all of the holds mentioned above or one of holds.

DEEP TISSUE MASSAGE

This is a slower massage that gets into the deeper layers of the fascia. It manually releases physical restrictions. Deep tissue massage helps break up scar tissue from previous injuries. Scar tissue is often sticky and clumpy and needs to be worked out. Ideally, you will find a therapist you can communicate with, so the pressure isn't too much or too little. Steer clear of massages that just hurt. For example, I went to a therapist once who I was told was good because she had deep pressure. She used her elbows to dig and although this felt good in moments, it hurt when she ran her elbows over my bones. Bone on bone is not good! If someone is digging an elbow into your spine or into your shoulder blade and not into the muscles surrounding the spine and shoulder blade, stop the massage. They don't know what they are doing, and you don't need to suffer for an hour.

REFLEXOLOGY

This modality focuses for the entire hour on the feet and sometimes the head and hands. The massage therapist applies pressure to specific points, and it affects the entire body. People who specialize in this are knowledgeable about which points on the feet and hands correlate with the rest of the body. This is a great option if you're uncomfortable with the idea of someone giving you a full-body massage. I was never interested in massaging people's feet or in having mine massaged until I took a reflexology class. After an hour of foot massage, I felt incredibly relaxed and a little nauseous. Each time I received it, I felt less nauseous and more at ease. It taught me to appreciate the subtle power of reflexology.

REIKI

This light-touch modality transfers healing light through the hands and into the client. Most of the time, it's done with the hands hovering above the body and clothes on. Some people include it into their oil massages as well. Many practitioners focus on symbols and various techniques to bring more light into the body and relieve pain in the physical, emotional, mental, and spiritual body. With light touch modalities like Reiki, you're never worried about someone applying too much pressure or moving the body in an abrupt way. You might think twice if the energetics of the massage feel off though, as sometimes two people don't vibe, and that's not going to help you heal.

Reiki has many levels of certification, the same way CranioSacral, and yoga does. Someone who has a Reiki one certification, such as myself, learns where to place their hands, how to connect to the light within and transfer it, and in the process they are attuned, which means a Reiki Master opens them up to receive the healing light from Reiki.

The first level of any certification is the tip of the iceberg. It gives the practitioner a landing place to begin the practice, but if you're drawn to Reiki as the main healing therapy, I recommend finding someone with more experience in that area. This does not necessarily mean they have to have more certifications, although education is always helpful. Some people are born with the gift to heal. For example, when I was in a CranioSacral training, I remember one woman putting her hands on my head and my whole body tingled with light. Keep in mind that this was a three day training, and I worked with over 20 people, but this one woman had a healing touch. When I asked her if she was Reiki certified, she said no, but everyone kept asking her that question. She was born with the gift, and sometimes that's the most important experience someone can have in the healing arts world.

ROLFING

This modality involves deep structural integration. The main focus is on relieving constricted fascia. When you see a Rolfing therapist, he will have you stand and walk around in your bra and underwear. He will check out your movement patterns before and after each massage. Generally the therapist requires you go through a 10 session protocol. Each massage targets a specific area of the body, and the entire hour is spent massaging that area open. Rolfing is given with deep pressure. If you're not a fan of deep work, check with the therapist before you get started to make sure he or she is comfortable adjusting the amount of pressure. Some Rolfers are known for going very deep work and not backing off. When I went through the ten sessions, which were designed to free restrictions trapped in various regions of the body, I worked with a woman who communicated with me as she applied pressure. She went up to my edge of comfort, but never beyond it. In the 10 sessions, I got more connected to other parts of my body. I learned that my neck wasn't tight just because of my neck and that it was all connected. The most beneficial gift I got from our sessions was learning to walk with my eyes lifted, rather than staring at the ground. This helped my neck tremendously!

SHIATSU MASSAGE

This is traditionally done on the floor or on a low table. Be sure to wear comfortable clothes during the massage. The therapist compresses points along the meridians and helps open the channels with a deeper touch. The same meridian points are used in Acupressure; the difference is this is more of a manual compression, rather than a light touch.

SOMATIC EXPERIENCING

Someone who is certified in somatic experiencing may or may not be a licensed psychologist. There is a difference between a Somatic

Therapist/Psychologist and someone certified in Somatic Experiencing. I worked with a woman who was a massage therapist, CranioSacral Therapist, and Certified Somatic Experiencing Practitioner. She helped me discover resources that calmed my nervous system before diving into traumatic events from the past. Then she used these resources to bring me into my body and the room whenever I started to get triggered. She was very skilled in her approach, and the bonus was sometimes she'd give me CranioSacral therapy or light massage. Many people use bodywork, breathwork, dance, and meditation to support healing. My Cognitive Behavioral Therapist uses Somatic Therapy techniques as a way to keep me body-centered and to stay connected to my mind and body. Be sure that whoever you choose to work with feels safe, kind, and easy to communicate with. If there is touch involved, it's important to have open dialogue with the practitioner, especially if you've had previous sexual assault. Be sure they are qualified and comfortable working with you, and if not, see if they can refer you to someone else.

SPORTS MASSAGE

Sports massage includes proprioceptive neuromuscular facilitation (PNF). This method stretches muscles to maximize their flexibility and is performed with a massage therapist or trainer who helps the client contract and relax specific muscles using various stretches. Sports massage is great for injury rehab and often includes trigger point therapy. I learned about sports massage in school for a 100 hours or so, but most of the learning I've gotten has come from working with people and helping them achieve results.

SWEDISH MASSAGE

This modality involves lots of slow strokes back and forth. It is a full body massage that is performed with the draping of sheets. The client gets undressed to their comfort level, and the therapist only reveals the part of the body they will be working on. If the client chooses to be fully naked, some therapists will undrape and work on the gluteus, or buttock, muscles. In the beginning of receiving massage, I would fully unrobe, and my first therapist worked on the gluteus muscles over the sheet. When I tried out someone new, they undraped my gluteus and didn't work over the sheets as I was used to. I held my breath the whole time he worked on them, terrified. What if he undraped my breasts next, or something else? I wish I had known ahead of time that this technique was a part of Swedish massage. Now you know. Some therapists will work over the sheets, and some with the sheets pulled to reveal the gluteus muscles. It doesn't mean they are going to try any funny business. You can relax. Overall, Swedish massage is incredibly relaxing! It can be given with a light, medium, or deep touch.

THAI MASSAGE

This is practiced on the floor with comfortable clothes on. It is similar to Shiatsu, but focuses more on joint mobilizations than acupressure points. The intention is to give with loving kindness. There are generally a lot of yummy stretches, and I've often heard it called "the lazy person's yoga." If you're someone who likes the idea of yoga, but can't bring yourself to practice it, this is a good place to start. Get your joints mobilized with the help of someone else and slowly increase your flexibility. If you're looking for a massage therapist to come to your home this is a great option. You don't need a table, just a cozy rug or cushion on the floor.

TUI NA

This is a fast-paced tapping, circling, jostling, or full-body sweeping. I've never experienced a full hour of this. It's usually given at the beginning or end of a massage or Acupuncture appointment. This kind of massage releases stagnant chi that gets locked up. My personal favorite is when a practitioner creates rhythmic karate chops to the top of the shoulder, right where most people hold tension, and the entire trapezius muscle relaxes. The first time a practitioner did this to me, I nearly melted on the table. All of the tension I held in my neck and shoulders didn't know what to do. It couldn't hold on, it couldn't tighten, so it just slowly let go.

AFTER A MASSAGE

Take notes before and after each massage, either mentally, in a voice memo, or on paper.

- Is your range of motion better or the same after the session?
- Has your stress level lowered?
- How long do the effects of the massage last?
- What did you enjoy about the massage?
- What would you like more of in the next session?
- Can the therapist accommodate your needs?
- Did you feel relaxed during the massage?
- Do you feel a sense of trust with the therapist?

CHAPTER 12

MOVEMENT RESOURCES

ASHTANGA YOGA

Ashtanga yoga is one of the most popular types of yoga being offered in yoga studios. It involves flowing with the breath, often with a lot of sun salutations where you will hold plank, downward facing dog, upward facing dog, and various other postures.

FELDENKRAIS

This kind of movement is sometimes incorporated into massage. I don't practice it, but I've had it done on me, and it feels very relieving. It involves feeling tension in the joints, applying rotation to them, and moving with the body in a slow and methodical way.

FOUNDATION TRAINING

Foundation Training is a series of body-weight exercises that activate your posterior muscle chain, anchors the hips, decompresses the spine, and teaches you to take the burden of supporting the body out of your joints and put it where it belongs: in your muscles. No matter your age or fitness level, Foundation Training puts you on the path to wellness. It is a great movement tool created by a chiropractor, Eric Goodman. This method helped me move out of chronic low back pain when I was commuting all over the Bay Area. It is a very specific sequence of postures that help you move better and perform better. There are foundation trainers all over the world, and if you have the opportunity to train with one, go for it!

FUNCTIONAL MOVEMENT PERSONAL TRAINER

This kind of personal trainer might have a functional movement certification from a company that specializes in Functional Movement, or they likely have an accumulation of the movement modalities referenced here. Most trainers who are certified in Foundation Training are teaching functional movement. I've found many Chiropractors and Physical Therapists are starting to work with personal trainers who specialize in functional movement.

IYENGAR YOGA

Iyengar Yoga focuses specifically on alignment. It can feel slow, especially if you are used to flowing through Sun Salutations, but it's a great place to start. One major breakthrough for my head and neck alignment was while holding plank in an Iyengar class. I'd held plank hundreds of times, maybe even thousands, never with confidence, nor with strength, most of the time I practiced on my knees in modified plank, looking toward my belly button.

Then I found a small Iyengar Yoga class in Pleasure Point, California. The instructor placed a foam roller along my spine and told me to connect the back of my head and my sacrum to the roller at the same time. Something clicked in my head and neck. For the first time, I felt what all the strong people holding planks must have been feeling all those years in flow yoga classes. Iyengar Yoga is great at using props to get your body into positions you can't seem to find on your own.

PILATES

Pilates came out of rehab. The machines and equipment used during sessions helps people to awaken muscles that have been injured or are asleep for some reason. Pilates focuses a lot on strengthening the pelvic floor muscles and is tremendous for many things, specifically pelvic floor rehab.

RESTORATIVE YOGA

Restorative yoga involves the use of many props. It's very common to only practice a few postures during a one hour class. Time is spent getting the body into a fully supported stretch that will both open the body and allow it to drop into deep relaxation. The benefits of holding supported postures and giving the nervous system a chance to relax from everyday stresses is a wonderful place to start.

THERAPEUTIC YOGA

Therapeutic yoga places an emphasis on breath as most yoga does; however, this kind of breath practice can be adapted to help an individual balance their emotional states. The kind of therapeutic yoga I studied was from the Structural Yoga lineage with Mukunda Styles. My teacher studied under him for years, and she passed on his teachings to myself and many other students. Structural yoga teaches the student how to strengthen, open, and mobilize the joints through the practice of the joint freeing series. Another well known form of Therapeutic yoga is Vini-Yoga. Therapeutic yoga focuses on optimizing the function of the body, not as much on how a pose is "supposed" to look.

TRX TRAINING

This is a way to strength train by using the weight of your own body. There are ways to increase and decrease the difficulty level of every exercise. TRX stands for Total Body Resistance Exercise. It is a great place to begin strength training especially if you have no desire to use weights or gyms scare you. You can easily set one of these up in your home or go to a gym that has private TRX classes.

WEIGHT LIFTING

There are many moments along the fitness and wellness path that have made me very uncomfortable. Lifting weights is a great example of an exercise that most days I find maddening, but I do it because it makes me feel better after.

Weight training can be done with free weights, barbells, cable and seated machines, medicine balls, and in the beginning body weight exercises might be enough of a challenge. This technique will help you get stronger as a way to get out of pain. I highly recommend signing up with a personal trainer who can familiarize you with equipment and start you with a safe beginners program.

CHAPTER 12: MOVEMENT RESOURCES

AFTER WORKING WITH A HEALING PROFESSIONAL

Take notes before and after each session, either mentally, in a voice memo, or on paper.

- Is your range of motion better or the same after the session?
- Has your stress level lowered?
- How long do the effects of the session last?
- What did you enjoy about the session?
- What would you like more of in the next session?
- Can the professional accommodate your needs?
- Do you feel confident in their ability to help you?
- Do you feel a sense of trust with the professional?

BIBLIOGRAPHY

"Biomechanical vs. Biodynamic CranioSacral Therapy." *Lumen Natura*. Dec. 15, 2011. https://www.lumennatura.com/2011/12/15/biomechanical-versus-biodynamic-CranioSacral-therapy/

"Discover CranioSacral Therapy and SomatoEmotional Release." *Upledger Institute International*. https://www.upledger.com/therapies/

Spangler PhD, Dr. Diane. "Depression After a Concussion: Why You Feel This Way and How to Start Healing." *Cognitivefx*. May 23, 2022. https://www.cognitivefxusa.com/blog/depression-after-concussion-and-post-concussion-syndrome

The Biodynamic CranioSacral Therapy Association of North America. https://www.CranioSacraltherapy.org/

www.ingramcontent.com/pod-product-compliance
Lightning Source LLC
Chambersburg PA
CBHW070358240426
43671CB00013BA/2559